A Volume in The Laboratory Animal Pocket Reference Series

The Laboratory
GUINEA
PIG

The Laboratory Animal Pocket Reference Series

Editor-in-Chief
Mark A. Suckow, D.V.M.
Laboratory Animal Program
Purdue University
West Lafayette, IN

Advisory Board

B. Taylor Bennett, D.V.M., Ph.D.
Biologic Resources Laboratory
University of Illinois at Chicago
Chicago, IL

John Harkness, D.V.M., M.S., M.Ed.
College of Veterinary Medicine
Mississippi State University
Mississippi State, MS

Terrie Cunliffe-Beamer, D.V.M., M.S.
The Jackson Laboratory
Bar Harbor, ME

Roger P. Maickel, Ph.D.
Laboratory Animal Program
Purdue University
West Lafayette, IN

Published and Forthcoming Titles

The Laboratory Rabbit

The Laboratory Non-Human Primates

The Laboratory Mouse

The Laboratory Guinea Pig

The Laboratory Rat

The Laboratory Hamster and Gerbil

The Laboratory Cat

The Laboratory Small Ruminant

A Volume in The Laboratory Animal Pocket Reference Series

The Laboratory
GUINEA PIG

Lizabeth A. Terril, D.V.M., M.S.

Purdue University
Laboratory Animal Program
West Lafayette, Indiana

Donna J. Clemons, D.V.M., M.S.

Diplomate ACLAM
Covance Laboratories, Inc.
Madison, Wisconsin

Editor-in-Chief
Mark A. Suckow, D.V.M.

CRC Press
Boca Raton   Boston   New York   Washington, D.C.   London

Photographs by Robert K. Werberig and Dr. Robert L. Hall.
Illustrations by Michael G. Tashwer.

Acquiring Editor: Marsha Baker
Project Editor: Helen Linna
Cover design: Denise Craig
PrePress: Kevin Luong

Library of Congress Cataloging-in-Publication Data

Terril, Lizbeth A.
    The laboratory guinea pig/ Lizbeth A. Terril and Donna J. Clemons
        p.   cm. — (The laboratory animal pocket reference series)
    Includes bibliographical references and index.
    ISBN 0-8493-2564-1
    1. Guinea pig—research. 2. Biology— laboratory animals. I. Clemons,
Donna, J.. II. Title.   III. Series.
    BR749.H79G87 1997
    616'.0149—dc20
                                         97-89103
                                             CIP

dedication

L.A.T. I want to thank my parents, Emmet and Virginia Terril and Patsy and Walter Owsley, for their guidance, support, and encouragement; my grandparents, Walter and Grace Terril and Roy and Ruby Buckler, for their inspiration, and last, but most important, my son, Brian, for his support and expert help. I also wish to thank Dr. Joseph E. Wagner and the University of Missouri for use of their slide collection and my colleagues at Purdue University who have helped make this endeavor possible.

D.J.C. My thanks to several colleagues for their help and patience that allowed me to have a part in this project. In particular, my appreciation to Mr. Mike Taschwer for putting his exceptional talents and hard work into the preparation of illustrations for this book; to Dr. Cindy Cary for her support of this project; and to Dr. Bob Hall for his expertise in photography. Last, but most importantly, thanks to my husband, Mark, for his endless encouragement and support of my career.

preface

The use of laboratory animals, including guinea pigs, continues to be an important part of biomedical research. In many instances, individuals performing such research are responsible for animal facility management, animal husbandry, regulatory compliance, and performance of technical procedures directly related to the research project. To help meet these responsibilities, this handbook was written to provide a quick reference source for investigators, technicians, and animal caretakers charged with the care and/or use of guinea pigs for research, teaching, or testing. It should be particularly valuable to small institutions or facilities lacking a large, well-organized animal resource unit and to individuals who need to conduct research on guinea pigs for the first time.

This handbook is organized into six chapters: "Important Biological Features" (Chapter 1), "Husbandry" (Chapter 2), "Management" (Chapter 3), "Veterinary Care" (Chapter 4), "Experimental Methodology" (Chapter 5), and "Resources" (Chapter 6). Basic information and common procedures are presented in detail. Other information regarding alternative techniques or details of procedures and methods which are beyond the scope of this handbook is referenced extensively so that the user is directed toward additional information without having to wade through a burdensome volume of detail here. In this sense, this handbook should be viewed as a basic reference source and not as an exhaustive review of the biology of the guinea pig.

The last chapter, "Resources," provides the user with lists of possible sources and suppliers of additional information, guinea pigs, feed, sanitation equipment, cages, and veterinary and research supplies. The lists are not exhaustive and do not imply endorsement of listed suppliers over suppliers not listed. Rather, these lists are meant as a starting point for users to develop their own lists of preferred vendors of such items. Also provided is a list of vendors of cages and research and veterinary supplies and contact information for these suppliers.

A final point to be considered is that all individuals performing procedures described in this handbook should be properly trained. The humane care and use of guinea pigs is improved by initial and continued education of all personnel and will facilitate the overall success of programs using guinea pigs in research, teaching, or testing.

the authors

Lizabeth A. Terril, D.V.M., is a laboratory animal veterinarian at Purdue University in West Lafayette, Indiana. She joined the University in 1993.

Dr. Terril earned her degree of Doctor of Veterinary Medicine from Oklahoma State University in 1988. She completed a residency in laboratory animal medicine at the University of Missouri in 1991 and remained as an Instructor in the Department of Veterinary Pathology until 1993. She also earned a Master of Science degree in laboratory animal medicine from the University of Missouri.

Dr. Terril is an active member in the national, Indiana Branch, and District 5 American Association for Laboratory Animal Science, and West Central Indiana Veterinary Medical Association. She is also a participating member of the American Society for Laboratory Animal Practitioners, and Laboratory Animal Management Association. Dr. Terril's research interests include the neurologic effects of nutritional deficiencies.

Donna J. Clemons, D.V.M., is clinical veterinarian for the laboratory animal medicine group of Covance Laboratories, Inc., Madison, Wisconsin.

Dr. Clemons earned the degree of Doctor of Veterinary Medicine from the University of Missouri in 1989, and completed a residency and Master of Science degree in laboratory animal medicine at the University of Missouri in 1992. She is a Diplomate of the American College of Laboratory Animal Medicine.

Dr. Clemons joined the staff of Covance Laboratories in 1992 and is responsible for the veterinary care of multiple species of animals. Her other duties include scientific assistance for studies, training and education, regulatory compliance, and program review. She is a member of the American Association for Laboratory Animal Science and an active participant in local branch activities.

contents

1 IMPORTANT BIOLOGICAL FEATURES   1

Introduction   1

Breeds   2

Behavior   6

   Individual Behavior   6

   Social Behavior and Communication   7

   Aggression and Reproductive Behavior   8

Anatomic and Physiologic Features   9

   External Anatomy   9

   Dentition   10

   Skeletal System   10

   Hemolymphatic System   12

   Gastrointestinal System   14

   Respiratory System   15

   Urogenital System   15

   Miscellaneous Unique Physiologic Features and
   Normative Values   19

      Hematology   19

      Cardiovascular and Respiratory Function   22

      Miscellaneous Physiologic and Anatomic Features   23

      Reproduction   23

2 HUSBANDRY   27

Housing   28

Environmental Conditions   35

Environmental Enrichment   37

Nutrition   39

Sanitation   41

Transportation   45

Record Keeping   46

3 MANAGEMENT   49

Regulatory Agencies and Compliance   49
  The U.S. Department of Agriculture   49
  The National Institutes of Health/Public Health Service   50
  The U.S. Food and Drug Administration and the
  Environmental Protection Agency   50
  Association for Assessment and Accreditation
  of Laboratory Animal Care International   50
Institutional Animal Care and Use Committee   51
Occupational Health and Zoonotic Diseases   53
Animal Health Monitoring Program   55

4 VETERINARY CARE   57

Basic Veterinary Supplies   57
Physical Examination of the Guinea Pig   58
Quarantine   59
Clinical Signs of Illness in Guinea Pigs   60
Common Clinical Problems   60
  Vitamin C Deficiency   61
  Bordetella bronchiseptica   62
  Streptococcus pneumoniae   64
  Cervical Lymphadenitis   65
  Antibiotic Toxicity   66
  Pregnancy Toxemia   67
  Salmonellosis   67
  Alopecia   69
  Malocclusion   73
  Protozoal Diseases   74
  Viral Diseases   75
  Pododermatitis   77
  Conjuctivitis   78
General Treatment of Disease   78
Disease Prevention through Sanitation   80
Anesthesia and Analgesia   80
  Principles of General Anesthesia   81
  Characteristics of Commonly Used
  Injectable Anesthetics   81
  Principles of Gas Anesthesia   84
  Characteristics of Commonly Used Gas Anesthetics   86
  Principles of Local Anesthesia   87

Sedation and Tranquilization of Guinea Pigs   88
Analgesia   88
Perianesthetic Management   89
Aseptic Surgery   92
Postsurgical Management   93
Euthanasia   94

5 EXPERIMENTAL METHODOLOGY   97
Restraint   97
Manual Restraint   97
Restraint Devices   99
Sampling Techniques   99
Blood Collection   99
Urine Collection   109
Milk Collection   110
Compound Administration Techniques   110
Intravascular   110
Intramuscular   113
Subcutaneous   114
Intraperitoneal   115
Intradermal   116
Oral   118
Intracerebroventricular   120
Aural — Middle Ear   120
Adjuvants   121
Safety Testing Procedures   121
Magnusson Maximization Test   122
Buehler Closed-Patch Sensitization Test   123
Guinea Pig Antigenicity (Anaphylaxis) Test   125
Sereny Test   125
Necropsy   125

6 RESOURCES   129
Organizations   129
Publications   132
Books   132
Periodicals   132
Electronic Resources   133
Animal Sources   134
Feed   135

Equipment   135
   Research and Veterinary Supplies   136
   Contact Information for Sources   136
Commercial Laboratories for Animal Health Monitoring   138

BIBLIOGRAPHY   139

INDEX   159

important biological features

introduction

Guinea pigs hold a place in human history that predates the European acquaintance with this small mammal. Long before cavies became synonymous with research subject, humans valued this animal as an important food source. To this day guinea pigs are considered a delicacy in many areas of South America, where domestic guinea pigs are allowed to roam and scavenge in and around the homes of the Indians.[1] The guinea pig's size, gentle nature, and coat variety make it a popular companion and hobby animal in the United States and other parts of the world. Researchers in the U.S. reported using over 360,000 guinea pigs in 1994 alone.[2]

By the 1500s, the domesticated guinea pig had been introduced to Europe. Spanish conquerors and sailors carried the small, docile animal throughout Europe, where it was bred for fancy and as pets for hundreds of years before its use in research. Research with guinea pigs is generally acknowledged to have started in the late-18th century, when Lavoisier used them in 1780 to measure heat production.[3] Since then, guinea pigs have been extensively used in studies of immunology, nutrition, otology, genetics, and infectious disease.[4,5]

It is uncertain where the misnomer "guinea pig" originated. Different names were used throughout the world, but it appears that some Europeans thought the animal a small pig from a foreign land. It has been suggested that the carcasses in the South American marketplace resembled small suckling pigs, but it's more likely that the vocalizations of the animals sounded like the squeals of pigs. This image is carried further in the common names used for the male and female, "boar" and "sow". "Guinea" may have been a distortion of the departure point from the new world, Guyana, or confusion because ships stopped on the coast of Africa on the way to Europe.[1] One source has suggested that the name may have come from the price (one guinea) of the animal in the English market.[6]

Taxonomically speaking, the guinea pig or more properly, *Cavia porcellus*, is a small mammal commonly accepted to be of the order Rodentia. Guinea pigs are further classified in the suborder hystricomorpha, or "porcupine"-like rodents, and the family Caviidae, tailless South American rodents with a single pair of mammae.[7] This traditional phylogenetic position, based on traditional morphological data, has been challenged in recent years due to modern studies of DNA and RNA sequences. Evidence based on the mitochondrial genome strongly supports the possible future inclusion of the guinea pig in a new mammalian order.[8]

The wild guinea pig is widespread in Argentina, Uruguay, Brazil, and other South American countries. Cavies live in variably sized groups in open grasslands, foraging on grasses and vegetables. Wild guinea pigs do not make nests or dig burrows, instead using natural shelters and burrows left by other animals.[9,10]

breeds

A number of stocks and strains of guinea pigs have been described, but only 5 are often used in research. The most common, the short-haired American or English guinea pig (Figure 1), is also the most popular laboratory and pet variety. Other typically used laboratory varieties include the Duncan-Hartley, Hartley, strain 2, and strain 13. English guinea pigs, Duncan-Hartley, and Hartley are outbred stocks. Duncan-Hartley

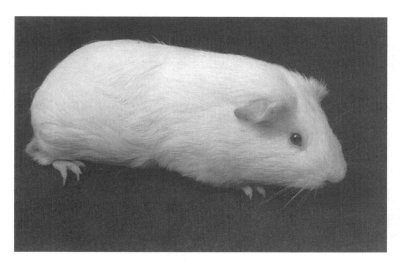

FIG. 1. An adult, albino, short-hair, Hartley strain guinea pig. The smooth, short-haired coat is found in the English and American Breeds.

and Hartley are short-haired albino animals and represent sub-lines of the English guinea pig, which has several coat colors. Inbred strains 2 and 13 are tricolor, with red, white, and black hair coats.[11]

Coat color is determined by the genotype at six main and several minor coat-color loci. The agouti locus produces the black coat color in the non-agouti mutant. The brown locus controls alteration from black to brown in the brown mutant. Four alleles are known for the albino locus, resulting in various degrees of dilution in coat and eye color. The laboratory albino guinea pig has the most extreme albino allele in addition to other dilution factors, resulting in an animal that has no pigment except on the ears. Three alleles at the extension locus are responsible for tortoise-shell coat patterns (partial extension) or yellow coat-color mutants (mutant e). The pink-eye locus also has three alleles; the pink-eye mutant causes dilution in both the retina and the coat. A white-spotting locus is responsible for the recessive white-spotting characteristic. Expression is determined by environmental and other genetic factors, and may result in an animal with a few white hairs, to a nearly completely white animal.[5]

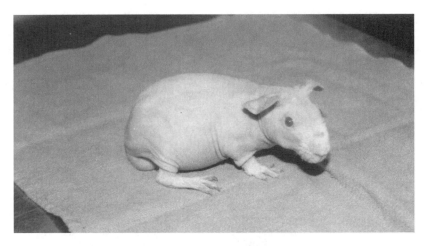

Fig. 2.   An adult, hairless guinea pig.

A number of other mutations have been identified that affect coat, color, skeletal structure, ear and circling behavior, enzymes, and antigen and disease resistance. Commercially available mutants include outbred hairless guinea pigs, an animal frequently used for dermatologic research (Figure 2).[12] A review of various mutants and guinea pig genetics may be found in Festing's chapter on guinea pig genetics in *The Biology of the Guinea Pig.*[13]

Breeds kept by fanciers but rarely in research include the Abyssinian and Peruvian (Figures 3 and 4). Abyssinian guinea pigs have short hair that grows in rosettes and whorls, giving them a rough, unkempt appearance. Peruvians have very long, silky hair that grows completely over their face and body, often touching the floor. These animals have a "rag mop" appearance, and require much grooming for the show ring. Animals prepared for show are sometimes found with their hair in curlers prior to judging.

Guinea pig fanciers are a small but devoted group of hobbyists that prefer to call their animals "cavies". Animals in a multitude of coat colors and patterns are exhibited by fanciers in organized shows. State fairs and 4-H shows are also places to see guinea pigs presented for exhibit and competition by their young owners.

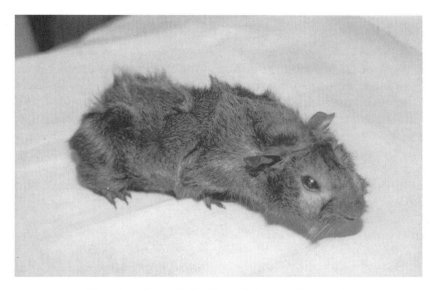

FIG. 3. An adult Abyssinian guinea pig

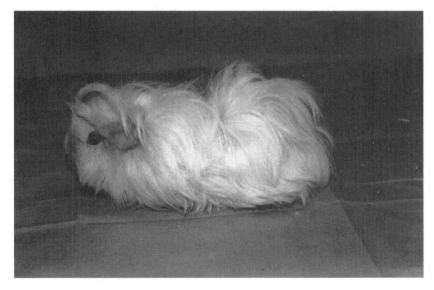

FIG. 4. An adult Peruvian guinea pig.

behavior

Most of the information about guinea pig behavior has come from observations of the animal in captivity. Wild cavy behavior is elusive. Individuals are most often observed scurrying to a hiding place. Wild colonies appear to live in loose, unorganized groups where a male dominates over several females. Two studies, by King in 1956 and Rood in 1972, have attempted to describe the behavior of guinea pigs under simulated natural conditions. [9,10] Many of these behaviors are reflected in the laboratory guinea pig.

Individual Behavior

Laboratory workers often view the guinea pig as a quiet, inactive animal but this may be a false impression based on an observed fear inhibition response of the animals. When placed in a quiet, comfortable environment, guinea pigs are almost continually active with no prolonged period of sleep. Singly housed guinea pigs are active 20 or more hours per day. Sleep, if it occurs at all, is for short periods or combined with a "sleep-walking" activity. [14] There is no distinct circadian pattern to the activity, but they appear to avoid intense light. In the wild, activity is greatest in early morning and evening, and in mid-day when the sky is overcast. [9,10]

Domestic guinea pigs share common behaviors with other laboratory rodents, but are unique in a number of ways. "Flight" in the guinea pig is characterized by intense "fleeing" with rapid, jerky rear limb motion continuing after running has ceased, and by "freezing", a response to sound. [15] "Fleeing", or "stampeding" as it is often called, is an example of contagious behavior, where an individual may trigger flight in the entire group after seeing movement. [9] Exploration of individuals and environments is slow and intermittent. Animals approach new individuals and objects with a stretched attention posture (face forward, body stretched), making contact with whiskers only. [15] Feeding is constant as long as food is available. [14] Feces are dropped anywhere. Elimination must be stimulated in young by the mother, who licks the anal region of her offspring. [9]

Social Behavior and Communication

Close proximity to other guinea pigs is well tolerated both at rest and when moving, the group providing a measure of security. The primary physical contact between adult guinea pigs is huddling, and may be more related to conserving heat than a desire for contact. There is little or no grooming between individuals except at mating and by mothers rearing young.[9,10] Social grooming, when it occurs, is performed by a female, who nibbles at the head and ears of the recipient.[10]

Olfactory signals play an important role in guinea pig social interactions. Scent marking with the large, perianal glands is made by dragging the perineal region across the ground. This behavior is often observed when animals are introduced to a new environment and when animals are in a mating encounter. Urine also has a communication function for the guinea pig. When a male approaches an unreceptive female he may throw his hindquarters against her while passing her, throwing a stream of urine towards her. This may serve to mark the female as one of his group. Unreceptive females also use urine, emitting a urine jet to repulse or distract persistent male investigations.

Guinea pig vocalizations have been identified as the primary means of communication within the species. Berryman has analyzed the frequency range and duration of guinea pig calls, identifying and naming at least 11 distinct vocalizations, each heard in specific situations.[16]

Exploratory behavior is often associated with the "chutt" and "putt", short duration sounds of varying frequency. "Chutter" and "whine" vocalizations are chains of sounds heard during (chutter) and after (whine) pursuit situations, such as males fighting or females courted by males. A "whistle" or "low whistle" is a longer call with a distinct rise in pitch. Guinea pigs use whistles when separated from each other, and when anticipating the arrival of food. Whistles may be single or repeated in long bouts. A rumbling, low-frequency "purr" and "drrr" (a very short purr) is heard when guinea pigs are seeking close physical contact. Young will purr when they wish to nurse, courting males and receptive females will purr, and hand-reared guinea pigs will purr when handled or fed. Injured and cornered animals will respond with "screams" or "squeals". Screams are not often heard in the laboratory, usually occurring in fights between unfamiliar animals. The sounds are shrill and harsh, and cover a large frequency range. The squeal is a similar sound, but short and sharp, in response to a transient or accidental injury. "Tweets" are soft sounds of ascending followed by descending frequency, heard when mothers stimulate young to defecate.[16,17]

Aggression and Reproductive Behavior

Aggression is less common and less severe in domestic *Cavia porcellus* than in their wild counterparts, but has many similarities. Aggressive actions and postures can be both offensive or defensive in nature. Mating privileges, space, and food are the primarily stimuli for aggressive interactions. Most aggression is between males, but actual fighting is rare. Females, even when newly introduced, will usually ignore each other, and are never attacked by the alpha male.[9,10]

Attend postures, a frozen position with the front legs extended, and eyes and ears forward, are seen in response to a potential threat. An aggressor may then approach with a head-thrust, where the head is jabbed forward repeatedly but does not contact the other animal. Adult animals use the head-thrust toward juveniles; females may use it defensively to repulse a male. Stand-threats occur when two unfamiliar animals, or animals with a disputed hierarchy, approach each other. After attending, each will assume a broadside body position, curving the rump towards the other individual. Both exhibit piloerection of the dorsal hair, making them appear larger. They may evert the rectum and tooth chatter while posturing. A leaping attack-lunge may follow with biting and clawing. If one of the animals chooses to flee, a chase may ensue.[9]

Defensive aggression is rare, mostly involving attempts by an unreceptive female to repulse a male. Females may whirl to face an investigating male, or kick back at him. The female will back into an unwelcome male with the perineum raised and back arched, then release a jet of urine towards his face.[9,10] When approached by a dominant animal, some subordinates will exhibit a head-up stance, a purely defensive action which is usually followed by a retreat. The animal throws the head back so that the nose is pointed straight up in the air. Males have been observed giving this response to defensive aggression.[10]

Adult males are attracted by estrous females and females in late gestation. In the presence of other subordinate males, the alpha male will guard these females aggressively. A male will investigate and court females with anogenital nuzzling and licking, purring, and swaying side to side rhythmically. Some will "rump" a female by throwing his hindlegs over her back while urinating. Receptive females will assume a lordosis posture with the pudendum raised, allowing the male to mount. The male clasps the female with his forepaws while rapidly thrusting. Ejaculation is accompanied by a drawing in of the flanks.[10] After copulation both male and female will groom; the male may drag his perineum on the ground.

Parturition occurs after a 58 to 75 day gestation, and may occur at any time of day. Labor is short, taking only five minutes from the start of labor until the first pup is born. Females may pull young with their teeth, then grasp and lick them clean. Fetal membranes are usually consumed, often with the help of other adult guinea pigs.[10] The precocial young begin to crawl toward their mother within minutes, and before they are one day old are usually walking, eating, and grooming. The mother passively allows nursing, and further maternal attention is limited to anogenital grooming.[18] Young will follow their mother, or less often, other adults who tolerate them. Fostering is common as domestic guinea pigs do not appear to discriminate well between their own offspring and other juveniles. Guinea pigs begin to nibble forage and solid food within the first few days of life, and are typically weaned around three weeks of age.[9,10]

anatomic and physiologic features

Cooper and Schiller's *Anatomy of the Guinea Pig* provides detailed information about all aspects of guinea pig anatomy.[19] Unique and important physiologic and anatomic features of the guinea pig include:

External Anatomy

- The guinea pig is a short, squat animal with a blunt head and short neck. The body is square with a rounded, tailless rump. Males are generally larger than the females.

- Both sexes have a single pair of abdominal mammae.

- Prominent mystacial vibrissae (whiskers) are present, with six parallel rows above the upper lip. Also present are mental vibrissae (under the chin), nasal vibrissae (on the dorsolateral nose), and supraorbital/infraorbital vibrissae (rostral/dorsal and inferior to the eye).

- The mouth is triangular with a split upper lip.

- External ears are large, oval, and sparsely haired.

- Cavia have four toes on the front foot but only three on the rear foot. Foot soles are hairless with well-defined footpads.

- The female perineum (Figure 5) has a single pair of lateral labia. Slightly protruding, the urethral orifice is located cranial to the prepuce of the clitoris. The U-shaped vaginal orifice is located in the center of the perineum and is bordered ventrally by the perineal sac, separating the vaginal opening from the anus. Filled with oily secretions, the perineal sac is a pouch of skin containing two perineal glands.

- Male guinea pigs (Figure 6) have large, prominent lateral scrotal swellings containing the testes. The urethra is the most cranial orifice, covered by the folded skin of the prepuce. Caudal to the urethral orifice, a longitudinal cleft covers the opening of the perineal sac and the anus.

Dentition

- All teeth are open-rooted and continuously growing.

- Adult guinea pigs have 20 teeth.

- Dental formula is 2 (1/1 incisors, 0/0 canines, 3/3 premolars, and 1/1 molars).

Skeletal System

- A complete zygomatic arch is found in the guinea pig, a distinguishing characteristic of the hystricomorph rodents.

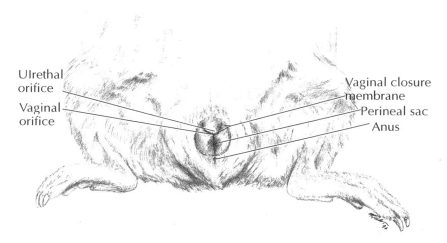

Ulrethal orifice

Vaginal orifice

Vaginal closure membrane

Perineal sac

Anus

FIG. 5.   External anatomy of the adult female guinea pig. Note the vaginal closure membrane.

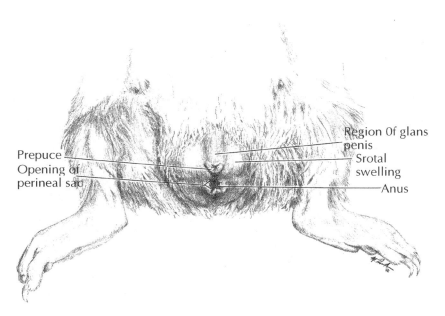

Prepuce
Opening of perineal sac

Region 0f glans penis

Srotal swelling

Anus

FIG. 6.   External anatomy of the adult male guinea pig.

- Vestigial clavicles are also present.

- Males have an os penis.

- The vertebral column is comprised of 34 to 38 vertebrae. Seven cervical vertebrae are followed by 13 to 14 thoracic vertebrae, which carry the 13 to 14 rib articulations. The first 6 pairs of ribs are true ribs, articulating with the sternum; ribs 7 to 9 are "false ribs", ribs that do not attach directly to the sternum, and articulate with the 6th rib cartilage. Ribs 10 to 14 are floating ribs which do not join the sternum. The last one or two pairs of ribs may be cartilaginous. Six lumbar vertebrae, 2 to 3 fused sacral vertebrae, and 4 to 6 caudal vertebrae complete the spinal column.

- Separate pelvic ox coxae fuse at around two weeks of age, but the connection remains cartilaginous in most animals. This symphysis will soften and degenerate in females beginning two weeks prior to parturition, allowing a wide separation to accommodate the birth of large fetuses.

Several anatomic features differentiate the guinea pig from other familiar laboratory rodents. While most structures are similar enough to other mammals in appearance to easily locate and identify, a few are worth mentioning for their inherent differences (Figure 7).

Hemolymphatic System

- The spleen is located in a similar position to that of other mammals and is broad and irregular in shape. Microscopically it consists of lymphatic tissue, arranged around small arteries, and is actually a hemolymph node.

- The thymus lies entirely within the neck of the guinea pig and consists of two, elongated oval lobes arranged on each side of the ventral midline. These structures are prominent in immature animals. Involution of the organ occurs as the animal ages, with mostly fatty tissue remaining by 12 months of age. Hassall's corpuscles, organizations of epithelial cells, are found within the thymus.[20]

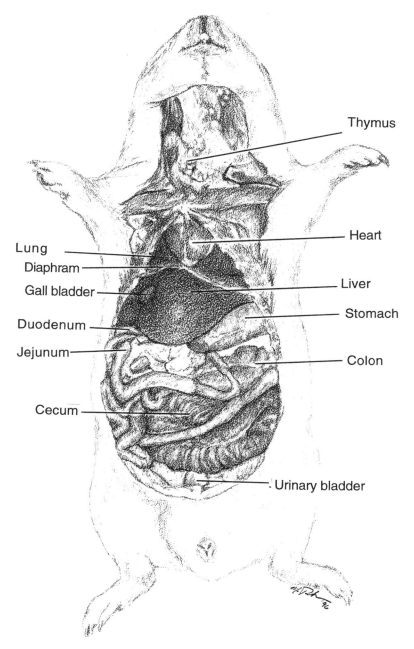

Fig. 7. Internal anatomy of the guinea pig. Note the cervical thymus, small thoracic cavity, and large cecum.

> **Note:** The cervical location of the thymus has made the guinea pig a popular model for immunological studies because it is easily accessed and removed.

- Lymph nodules and Peyer's patches are present throughout the small intestine, becoming more numerous towards the distal portion.

Gastrointestinal System

- The stomach lies in the left cranial portion of the abdomen, and contacts the left lobe of the liver. There are four regions: the cardia, fundus, body, and pylorus. The **cardia** is a small area surrounding the esophagus as it passes through the stomach wall. The **fundus** is large, pouching out left and cranial to the cardia. The smaller **body** of the stomach lies to the right of the fundus and leads into the thick-walled **pylorus**, which connects the stomach to the small intestine. The inner surface of the cardia and fundus is smooth; rugae, wrinkles, or folds, are present in the body and pylorus. There is no keratinized portion to the gastric mucosa, which is entirely glandular in nature.

- Three functional areas of the small intestine, duodenum, jejunum, and ileum, may be distinguished by location and microscopic differences, but cannot be identified by external landmarks. The entire small intestine is approximately 125 cm in length. The ileum ends with an infolding of the mucosa, the ileocecal papilla, at the entry to the cavity of the cecum.

- The cecum is the most characteristic feature of the guinea pig gastrointestinal tract. It is a large, thin-walled semicircular sac with numerous lateral pouches.

- Six liver lobes are usually identified in the guinea pig: right lateral, right medial, left lateral, left medial, caudate, and quadrate lobes.

- The biliary system drains into a common hepatic duct.

- The gallbladder is attached to a fossa in the quadrate lobe of the liver.

- A small cystic duct leads from the neck of the gallbladder to join the common hepatic duct, forming the common bile duct, a light-colored, pinkish-white structure, which in turn extends to the duodenum. The common bile duct enters the duodenum approximately 5 mm distal to the pyloric valve, terminating at the duodenal papilla.

- Sources disagree on whether the pancreatic duct joins the common bile duct or drains separately into the duodenum.[19,20]

Respiratory System

- The lungs are divided into seven lobes: four right lobes (cranial, middle, caudal, and accessory) and three left lobes (cranial, middle, and caudal).

Note: The bronchi are extremely histamine sensitive and prone to spasm during immediate hypersensitivity reactions. There are few distinguishing anatomical characteristics of this in the lungs.

- Prominent perivascular lymphoid nodules are found around branches of pulmonary arteries and veins in most guinea pigs, and tend to increase in size as the animal ages. Eventually these nodules can become large enough to be grossly visible at necropsy. The purpose of these nodules is not known.

Urogenital System

- Renal tubules are straight and give the renal medulla a rather striated appearance.

- The renal pelvis is large and characterized by a single papilla.

- Ureters drain the kidneys into a large, thin walled urinary bladder.

- The female urethra terminates at the urethral orifice, the most cranial orifice of the vulvar region.

- The female reproductive organs are the ovaries, oviducts, uterus, and vagina (Figures 5 and 8).

- The ovarian bursa is closed off from the peritoneal cavity except for a small cranioventral opening.

- The ovaries are yellowish, flattened organs that vary from smooth to nodular in appearance depending on the point in the reproductive cycle. Narrow, coiled oviducts lie lateral to the ovaries, and connect the ovary to the uterine horn.

- The bicornate uterus, a pink, Y-shaped organ, passes from the oviducts to the vagina. In the nongravid female, the organ lies dorsally within the peritoneal cavity. The uterus has two horns, a body, and a single cervix. During pregnancy, each fetus will appear as a single swelling in the uterine horns.

- The vagina is characterized by the vaginal closure membrane, a feature unique to the hystricomorph rodents. This membrane is perforate only at estrus and parturition.

- The male guinea pig reproductive system (Figures 6 and 9) is comprised of the penis, testes, epididymis, ductus deferens, vesicular glands, prostate, coagulating glands, and bulbourethral glands.

- The testes lie in shallow scrotal sacs on either side of the perinuem. Large, permanently open inguinal rings communicate with the peritoneal cavity, allowing the testes to also be found within the abdominal cavity (Figure 9).

- An intromittent sac, a structure unique to hystricomorphs, lies on the ventral aspect of the glans penis. During erection, the sac everts protruding two keratinaceous styles. The function of this anatomic feature is unknown.

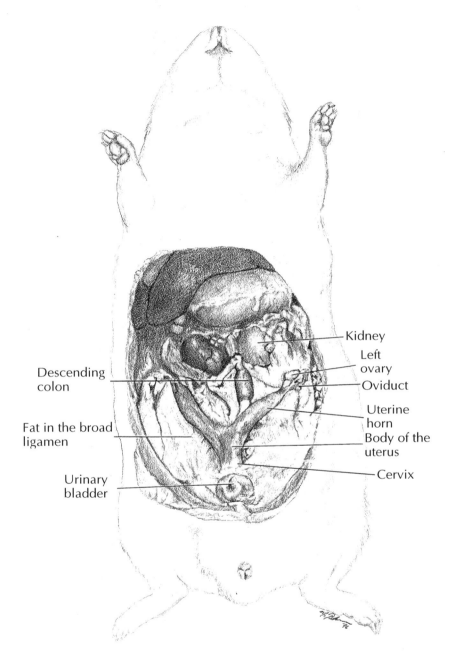

Fig. 8. Internal anatomy of the adult female guinea pig with identification of reproductive organs.

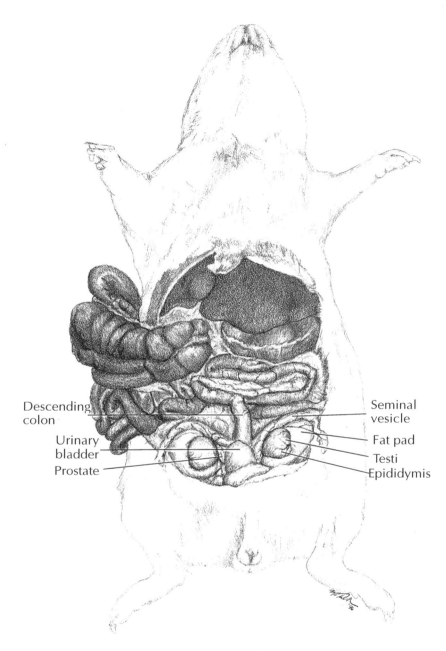

Descending colon

Urinary bladder

Prostate

Seminal vesicle

Fat pad

Testi

Epididymis

Fig. 9. Internal anatomy of the male guinea pig with identification of the reproductive organs.

TABLE 1. BASIC BIOLOGIC PARAMETERS OF THE GUINEA PIG

Parameter	Typical value	Reference(s)
Diploid chromosome number	64	21
Life span (years)	3–7	21
Body weight, adult male (g)	900–1000	22
Body weight, adult female (g)	700–900	22
Body surface area	9.5 (weight in g)$^{2/3}$	23
Body temperature (°C)	39.2 ± 0.7	24
50% Survival (months)	60	22
Food consumption (g/kg/day)	60	21
Water consumption (ml/kg/day)	100	21
GI Transit time (hours)	13–30	25
Urine pH	9	26

Miscellaneous Unique Physiologic Features and Normative Values

Relatively little research has focused specifically on defining the normal physiology of the guinea pig. Most normative data has been gleaned from papers on disease-oriented research. This section reviews several areas of guinea pig physiology and assembles potentially useful information relative to the use of the guinea pig as an animal model. Normative data for basic biologic parameters are summarized in Table 1, hematologic data in Table 2, clotting factor data in Table 3, clinical chemistry data in Table 4, cardiovascular and respiratory data in Table 5, and basic reproductive data in Table 6.

> **Note:** Guinea pigs exhibit a wide range of individual variation in hematologic parameters. Diet, age, physiologic status, breed, method of sample collection, and differences between laboratories all contribute to the degree of variation observed in the many published reports providing data on guinea pigs. It is necessary for each individual laboratory to establish normal values for their specific facility.

hematology

- Relative to other common laboratory species, such as the rat and mouse, the guinea pig has lower red blood cell numbers and a lower hemoglobin concentration, similar to the rabbit.[27]

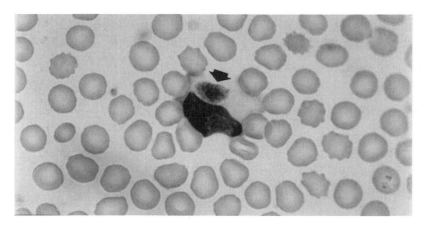

FIG. 10. Photomicrograph of a Kurloff cell surrounded by red blood cells. The Kurloff is a mononuclear leukocyte with an ovoid inclusion and is found in large numbers in pregnant females.

- The erythrocytes are quite variable in size.

- Guinea pig hemoglobin is similar to dog, rat, horse, rabbit and man in it's relatively high affinity for oxygen,[28] yet differs significantly from dog, rabbit, and man by being resistant to oxidation to methemoglobin.[29]

- Kurloff cells are a unique feature of the guinea pig leukon. The cell is a mononuclear leukocyte with round to ovoid inclusions that range from 1 to 8 um in size (Figure 10). The origin and function of the cell has not been proven, but most consider the spleen to be the primary source of these cells.[30] Mucopolysaccharides secreted from the cell make up the inclusion material.[31] Studies of the Kurloff cell have shown their numbers increase with elevations of estrogen and that the cells migrate to the placenta in pregnant guinea pigs,[32] leading to speculation that Kurloff cells function as a physiologic barrier protecting the embryos from sensitized lymphocytes and IgM.[33]

- Like humans, the guinea pig possesses a lymphomyeloid complex that is very mature at birth plus has a cervical thymus that is easily accessible for measurement and manipulation.[34] Also like man, treatment with steroids

TABLE 2.   HEMATOLOGIC VALUES OF THE GUINEA PIG

Parameter	Typical Value	Reference(s)
Red blood cell count (10^9/ml)	4.5–7.0	39
Packed cell volume (%)	37–48	40,41
Hemoglobin (g/100ml whole blood)	11.0–15.2	40
Red blood cell size (μm)	7.1–8.27	42,43
Red blood cell life span (days)	60–80	44
Mean cell volume (fl)	85–91	40
Mean cell hemoglobin concentration (%)	31.5 ± 0.59	40,45
Mean cell hemoglobin (pg)	25	46
Total leukocyte count (10^3/mm^3)	4.80 ± 5.5	41
Neutrophils (%)	31.3 ± 2.04	41
Lymphocytes (%)	64.6 ± 4.89	41,47
Eosinophils (%)	0–3	48
Monocytes (%)	0–7	48
Basophils (%)	0–2	48
Platelets (10^5/mm^3)	6.2 ± 0.12	49

TABLE 3.   CLOTTING FACTOR VALUES IN THE GUINEA PIG

Parameter	Typical Value	Reference(s)
One-stage prothrombin time (PT), seconds	25.3–29.16	37,49,50
Partial thromboplastin Time (PTT), seconds	13–49	49,51
Thrombin time, seconds	27.5–48.0	37
Factor II (Prothrombin) Iowa units	85–243	37,49
Factor V (labile factor) Units/100 mL plasma	55–140	37,51,52
Factor VII (stable factor) units/100 mL plasma	0–0.61	37,51
Factor VIII (antihemophilic factor) units/100 mL plasma	63–142	49
Factor IX (plasma thromboplastin) units/100 mL plasma	67–141	49
Fibrinogen (mg/100 mL plasma)	30–300	37,49,52

does not affect thymic physiology, causing the guinea pig to be considered a steroid resistant species.[35] The thymus is a major source of circulating lymphocytes, but by 12 months of age the thymus has involuted, and contains fat deposits.[36]

TABLE 4. CLINICAL CHEMISTRY VALUES IN THE GUINEA PIG

Parameter	Typical value	Reference(s)
Serum protein (g/dl)	5.0–5.6	39
Albumin (g/dl)	2.8–3.9	39
Globulin (g/dl)	1.7–2.6	39
Serum glucose (mg/d)	125 ± 13	39
Blood urea nitrogen (mg/dl)	8–28	53
Creatinine (mg/dl)	0.6–2.2	21
Total bilirubin (mg/dl)	0.3–0.9	21
Triglycerides (gm/dl)	0–145	53
Cholesterol (g/dl)	21–43	53
Serum calcium (mEq/dl))	4.64 ± 0.63	39
Serum phosphate (mEq/dl)	3.0–7.6	39
Magnesium (mg/dl)	2.3	39
Sodium (mEq/dl)	137.3 ± 11.4	39
Chloride (mEq/dl)	92.3 ± 10.4	39
Potassium (mEq/dl)	8.1 ± 1.6	39
Triiodothyroxine T_3 (pg/ml)	317	54
Total thyroxine (ng/ml)	45	53

- Guinea pig fibrinogen values fall within the normal range for human values.[37]

- Platelet function may more closely resemble humans than other species, particularly in regard to aggregation.[38]

Cardiovascular and Respiratory Function

Studies of guinea pig cardiovascular and respiratory physiology demonstrate that guinea pigs respond in a predictable manner to manipulations and environmental changes, even when there is no overt behavioral response. Normative values are given in Table 5.

- Animals respond with elevated heart rates to stimuli such as human handling, the presence of other animals, and novel objects. Animals accustomed to the various stimuli have heart rate increases of a lesser magnitude.

- Guinea pig electrocardiogram resembles that of humans, having easily identifiable *P, Q, R, S,* and *T* waves.[55] The basic rhythm is sinusal and regular. Guinea pigs, like humans, have a *T* wave that is distinctly separate from the *QRS* complex.[56] There is a large degree of individual variation within the species.[55,57]

TABLE 5.   CARDIOVASCULAR AND RESPIRATORY FUNCTION
            IN THE GUINEA PIG

Parameter	Typical value	Reference(s)
Heart rate (per minute)	229–319	58
Blood pressure (mm Hg avg)	76.7/46.8 anesthetized	59
Blood pressure (mm Hg)	80–94/55–58 unanesthetized	21
Respiratory rate (per minute)	42–104	60
Tidal volume (ml/kg)	2.3–5.3	60
Blood volume (ml/kg)	69.6	52
Marrow blood volume (ml/kg)	1.0–1.2	52
Plasma volume (ml/kg)	38.8	52

Miscellaneous Physiologic and Anatomic Features

- Guinea pigs lack central adrenergic neurons.[61]

- The guinea pig eye is similar in most general characteristics to that of other rodents. A retina with few vessels, clustered closely around the optic disk is a distinguishing feature.[62]

- Guinea pigs have been widely used in studies of anaphylaxis, and the role of histamine sensitivity in acute bronchospasm. Research focused on pulmonary function/structure in the guinea pigs has found them to be unique in having the majority (over 92%) of the pulmonary stretch receptors located in the small airways and pulmonary parenchyma.[63]

Reproduction

A wealth of data is available on the reproduction of the guinea pig, serving both researchers and producers of research animals. Some basic information concerning guinea pig reproduction has been summarized in Table 6.

Note: Guinea pigs are an important model for the study of reproductive biology, made even more useful by similarities to human reproductive biology. Like humans, guinea pigs have a long gestation period, spontaneous ovulation, and active corpora lutea. Polyestrous, nonseasonal cycling with visible estrus, and a fertile postpartum estrus further add to the usefulness of the guinea pig in the laboratory.

TABLE 6. REPRODUCTIVE FUNCTIONS OF THE GUINEA PIG

Parameter	Normal value	Reference(s)
Male breeding onset (g)	600–700 (3–4 mon)	22,64
Female breeding onset (g)	350–450 (2–3 mon)	22,65,66
Breeding duration (mon)	20	22
Cycle length (days)	15–19	5,67
Estrus duration (hours)	6–11	5
Gestation period (days)	58–75	5
Parturition length (minutes)	10–30	68
Litter size	2–5	22,69
Birth weight (g)	90–120	22,69
Weaning age (g)	150–200 (14–21 days)	5,22
Postpartum estrus	Fertile, 3.5 hours	21,68,70
Postpartum pregnancy rate (%)	60–80	21,68,70
Lactation length (days)	18–23	71
Peak lactation (days postpartum)	5–8	71

- Proestrus is often characterized by the behavioral signs of courting (swaying, pursuit of cage mates), and may last for up to 50 hours before estrus. The onset of estrus can also be detected by behavioral clues from the guinea pig. Females reliably exhibit the copulatory reflex, with lordosis, lowering the back, and elevation of the posterior.[72]

- The vaginal membrane, the epithelial structure sealing the vagina, will rupture just prior to the onset of estrus, and will stay open for approximately 2 days in mature sows, closing after ovulation.[73]

- Ovulation occurs approximately 10 hours after the onset of estrus, usually after the vaginal membrane has been open for 1 day.[72,74]

- Vaginal cytology may be used as a reliable indicator of the onset of estrus.[75]

- Fluid from the seminal vesicles of the male, with contributions from the anterior lobe of the prostate gland, coagulates almost immediately upon emission. In natural breeding, this material constitutes the copulatory plug, a feature generally found in rodent species. The plug fills the vagina and cervix, keeping sperm in, then falls out within a few hours.[76] Identification of this plug in the cage may be used to verify mating.

- Guinea pigs are frequently housed as a harem for breeding, one male with one to ten females. The females may be either left with the male for their entire reproductive life and the young removed at weaning or removed before parturition and returned to the harem after weaning.[21]

- Guinea pigs do not build nests.[21]

- Duration of gestation is variable, being inversely proportional to the number of fetuses. Long gestations and relatively mature young make the guinea pig a desirable subject for teratology studies.

Note: Rats, rabbits, and mice will abort their young once ovaries have been removed making the guinea pig a valuable model for the study of the endocrine control of human pregnancy.[77]

- Morphologically, the guinea pig placenta resembles that of the human.[65] The placenta is classified as a hemochorial type similar to the mouse, rat, rabbit, and human, with direct contact of the maternal blood supply and the fetal trophoblast.

- Fetuses may be palpated within the uterus at 4 to 5 weeks into gestation.[21]

- Unlike other species, the event which triggers parturition is not known. It does not appear linked to a drop in the progesterone level as in other species. During the last half of gestation, relaxin levels increase causing a relaxation of the pubic symphysis. As the symphysis softens, it separates, increasing the size of the birth canal.[78] A separation of 15 mm indicates parturition within 48 hours.[21]

Note: Some breeders feel that it is desirable to breed young sows on their first heat to maximize the separation of the pubic symphysis for later pregnancies.

- Young are precious at birth, with open eyes and ears, full hair coats, and teeth. They begin eating solid food during the first few days of life.[21] Nursing is not absolutely necessary to the survival of the young; 50% have been shown to survive without nursing.[79] However, nursing for 15 to 20 days greatly enhances survivability and body weight gains in the neonatal guinea pigs.

- Guinea pig milk differs from that of other rodents in it lacks short-chain fatty acids, and more resembles human and canine milk in this respect.[80] The milk contains about 4% fat, 8% protein, and approximately 77 calories per 100 grams.[81]

- Neonates may not nurse until 12 to 24 hours of age.[21]

- Guinea pig young should be weaned at 14 to 28 days of age or 150 to 200 g body weight.[21]

2

husbandry

Good husbandry is an essential component of a quality animal care program. Husbandry factors not only greatly influence the health and well-being of the research guinea pig, but also have the potential to affect the outcome of current and future research studies. Good husbandry programs/practices take into account not only the immediate surroundings of the guinea pigs (**microenvironment**), but also the larger environment of the room and facility (**macroenvironment**). The microenvironment includes aspects such as type of caging system, bedding, in the cage temperature and humidity, intensity of lighting in the cage, noise, cagemates, feed, and novel manipulative items; while the macroenvironment includes aspects such as room design, location of cage in the room and on the cage rack, room temperature and humidity, room illumination, noise, and animal care personnel. It is apparent that many of these factors are intertwined and affect both the micro- and macroenvironments of the research guinea pig.

The *Handbook of Facilities Planning* discusses in detail the many concerns and considerations necessary for the building of a good research animal facility and also the aspects of designing a good room for housing research guinea pigs.[82] The *Guide for the Care and Use of Laboratory Animals* contains a compilation of recommendations for guinea pig husbandry and management[83] and the Regulations of the Animal Welfare Act details principles which must be followed by persons using guinea pigs in research, teaching, and testing.[84] The contents of these documents regarding guinea pig use and care are included in the information presented in this and following chapters.

housing

The following items of the macroenvironment must be considered in the development of optimal guinea pig housing:

1. Location of the animal room within the facility.

   • This should be away from areas of excessive noise and vibration, such as cagewash equipment, dog and nonhuman primate housing, and computer equipment. Increased levels of noise and vibration have been documented to produce a physiologic stress response in guinea pigs.[85,86]

   • The room should be located in an area with easy access to the necessary sanitation equipment.

   • The caging equipment should easily move through doorways, around the room, and down the hallway(s).

   • Research personnel must be able to easily access the room.

2. The design of the individual room housing the research guinea pigs.

   • The room should provide enough space for the easy movement of personnel performing daily animal care tasks such as cage cleaning and changing.

   • The floor should slope toward the drain, but not so steeply to make it impossible to maintain stable guinea pig caging. A drain in the guinea pig room is not a necessity, but room maintenance is easier with one.

   • Many activities are facilitated by the presence of a sink with hot and cold water within the animal room.

3. Construction materials used within the facility and room.

    •   All surfaces of floors and walls must be able to withstand repeated disinfection procedures with the wall-floor junction being sealed and also impervious to these procedures.

    •   The floors should allow easy movement of equipment, but at the same time provide stable footing for animal care personnel.

    •   Doors should be able to withstand repeated disinfection procedures, while providing security for the guinea pigs housed inside.

4. Equipment to be maintained within the room.

    •   Mops and brooms, or any equipment necessary for the sanitary maintenance of the room.

    •   Animal care equipment necessary for the appropriate care of the guinea pigs.

    •   Necessary research equipment for the current study.

    •   All equipment maintained within the animal room must be kept out of the reach of the guinea pigs and stored in a manner that prevents clutter and facilitates sanitation.

Microenvironmental variables are as important, if not more so, to the appropriate housing of the guinea pig as are the previously discussed macroenvironmental factors. The caging system in which the guinea pig is housed should be of utmost concern. In the selection of appropriate caging, the following items must be considered:

1. The **size of the cage**, measured as floor area, must be large enough to accommodate the natural movements and body shape and size of the guinea pig. It should also accommodate the concurrent housing of multiple animals, breeding pairs or groups, and mothers with young. Table 7 lists the cage sizes required by the Animal Welfare Act[84] and the Guide for the Care and Use of Laboratory

TABLE 7.   CAGE SIZE FOR GUINEA PIGS

Body Weight (g)	Floor Space/Guinea Pig in² (cm²)	Interior Cage Height in (cm)
(350	60 (387.12)	7 (17.78)
>350	101 (651.65)	7 (17.78)
Nursing female with young	101 (651.65)	7 (17.78)

Animals[83] for housing guinea pigs and the information listed is summarized from these documents. The requirements for both are the same. It should be noted that even though cage size for guinea pigs is regulated, group housed animals frequently use just the cage space located along the periphery of the cage.[87]

2. Cage construction materials should provide a smooth, nonporous surface that is easy to clean, able to withstand repeated disinfection, resistant to corrosion, and strong enough to support and contain the guinea pig(s). Stainless steel and heavy-duty plastics meet these criteria and are the most frequently used materials for the construction of guinea pig cages. Figure 11 is an example of a standard plastic "shoebox" cage for guinea pigs.

3. The cage design should accommodate the normal behavioral and physiological needs of the guinea pig, including body temperature regulation, normal movement and postural adjustment, urination and defecation, and when necessary, reproduction. They should allow the animals to remain clean and dry, allow easy access to food and water, be free of sharp edges and projections, provide a secure environment that does not allow entrapment of the animal between opposing surfaces or within openings, and allow easy viewing of the guinea pig with minimal disturbance.[83,88]

   • Floors may be solid, slotted, or wire-mesh, When wire-mesh floors are used, care must be taken to ensure that the openings are big enough to allow urine and feces to pass through, yet small enough to prevent entrapment of the feet of the guinea pig. Guinea pigs are known to attain an adult weight of

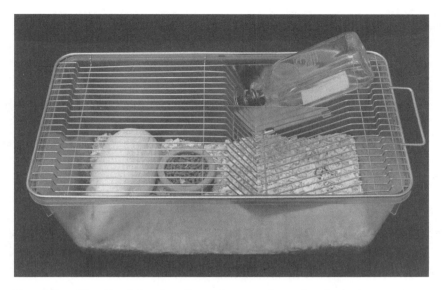

FIG. 11. Plastic "shoebox" caging system for housing guinea pigs. The cage allows easy access to feed and water and is easily cleaned.

up to 1 kg and have relatively small feet. The wire-mesh, if inappropriately sized, may contribute to the development of pressure sores on the plantar surface of the feet (pododermatitis) in the adult or broken legs in juveniles. Recommended mesh opening size is 75 × 12 mm.[88,89] Current recommendations indicate that solid-bottom cages with contact bedding are the preferred method of housing guinea pigs.[83]

- Due to the behavioral and anatomic attributes of the guinea pig, tops on cages are usually not necessary. Guinea pigs rarely jump and seldom climb. Figure 12 shows a rack of hard-plastic guinea pig cages, without tops, for group housing.

- Watering devices that may be used for guinea pigs include ceramic bowls, bottles attached to the cage exterior (Figure 13), and automatic watering systems (Figure 14). The stocky, short-necked build of a guinea pig may allow damage to the ventral neck

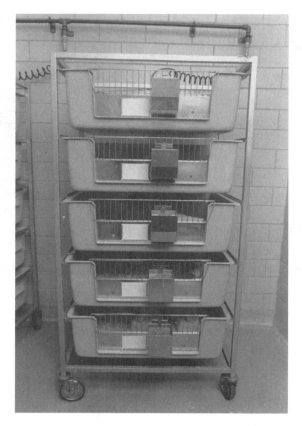

FIG. 12. Caging system for group housing guinea pigs composed of large, hard plastic and stainless steel cages, automatic watering system, stainless steel feeders, and cage card holders.

if inappropriate watering devices are used. Watering devices should be located well above the level of the bedding in the cage as guinea pigs like to "play " with their waterer and may flood their cage by placing bedding in the device. Automatic watering devices should have the valve located outside of the cage.[21] When selecting a watering device, it should be remembered that guinea pigs do not like, nor adapt well to new items in their environment, therefore, it may be necessary to train newly received guinea pigs to the watering system by holding them to the system and touching their mouth on the

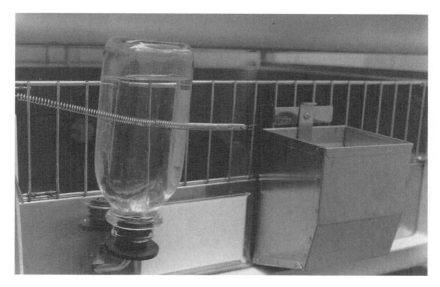

Fig. 13.   Individual guinea pig cage with attached water bottle.

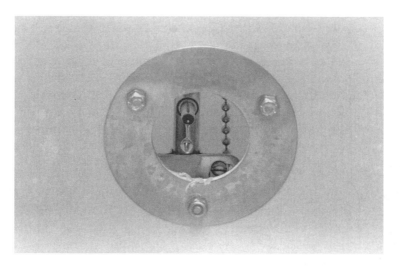

Fig. 14.   Automatic watering device found in the back of a guinea pig cage. Note that the valve is located outside of the cage.

water source a number of times each day for two to three days. Guinea pigs have been known to die of dehydration because they were unfamiliar with the watering device.[88]

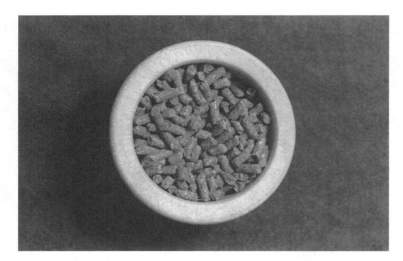

FIG. 15.   Ceramic feed bowl, containing pelleted guinea pig feed.

- Feed containers acceptable for guinea pigs include ceramic bowls (Figure 15 containing standard guinea pig feed) and feeders attached to the exterior of the cage. Guinea pigs rarely rise up on their hind legs, so feeding them in the rack in the top of the cage is not an acceptable method. The guinea pig also has a predilection for urinating, defecating, and nesting in bowls or crocks, therefore, a metal J-feeder attached to the outside of the cage is the preferred feeding method (see Figure 16). Automatic feeding devices have been developed for quantitative feeding studies.[90]

Bedding is frequently used in guinea pig housing. It may be used in direct contact with the animal, in the bottom of the cage, or indirectly, beneath hanging cages. Bedding materials used include paper products, corn cob products, and hardwood products (Figure 17). These materials may be shredded, chipped, ground, or pelleted. Softwood products are not used because they contain aromatic hydrocarbons that induce liver enzymes, increase the incidence of cancer, and may adversely affect research.[83,91] Whatever material is used, it should be almost dust free, since guinea pigs like to dig with their nose

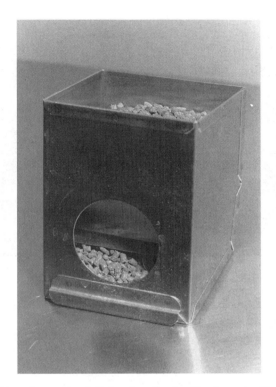

FIG. 16. Stainless steel J-feeder that attaches to the cage. The preferred feed container.

in the bedding and might get small particles into the lungs. Bedding that is too small can be easily eaten and/or may become impacted in the genital openings of the guinea pig and infertility may result.[92] The material should be absorbent to reduce moisture and odor in the cage. A study by Marshall et. al demonstrated that growing guinea pigs preferred a cage containing bedding over wire-mesh bottom cages.[93]

environmental conditions

Environmental conditions play an important role in the husbandry practices for maintaining research guinea pigs. The following environmental conditions should be closely monitored and controlled:

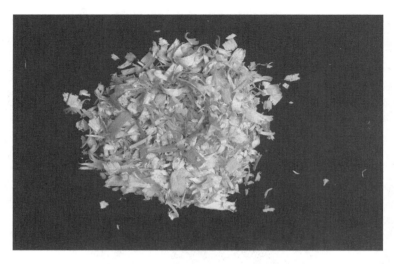

Fig. 17. Typical hardwood bedding, free of dust and contaminants. May be used within the guinea pig cage and beneath suspended cages.

1. Temperature plays an important role in guinea pig health. The stout, compact body of a guinea pig does not dissipate heat very well, therefore, they are very sensitive to changes in temperature and do not tolerate extreme heat very well. Environmental temperatures above 75 to 80°F may induce heat stress/stroke. The recommended temperature, measured via dry-bulb, for a guinea pig room is 64 to 79°F (18 to 26°C).[83]

2. Relative humidity is related to temperature and should be maintained at 30 to 70%.[83]

3. Illumination can influence the physiology, reproduction, and well-being of guinea pigs. The amount of light needed by an animal may be influenced by light intensity, duration of exposure, wavelength of light, time of light exposure, pigmentation of the animal, hormonal status, previous light exposure, age, sex, and genetic makeup. Lighting should be diffused through the entire room and provide enough illumination for personnel to easily perform daily husbandry tasks and easily observe the guinea pigs. Recommendations for appropriate illumination of guinea pig rooms include a 12 to 14 hour lights on with an associated

12 to 10 hour lights out cycle and an intensity of 325 lux (30 ft candles) at 1 meter above the floor.[83]

4. Ventilation of the guinea pig room should reduce odors, but not produce excessive drafts which are not well tolerated by guinea pigs. It is recommended that there be 10 to 15 fresh air changes per hour per room. Recirculation of room air may be acceptable if the air is filtered to remove potential airborne pathogens.[83,88] Ventilated racks and cages may also be used for adequate ventilation.

5. Noise within the animal room and surrounding area should be kept to a minimum. Guinea pigs are easily startled by loud noises and may "stampede" or "freeze".[9,15,85,86]

Note: Daily fluctuations in environmental conditions should be kept to a minimum.

Note: Environmental conditions within the room may differ from those within the cage, therefore, the microenvironment of the cage should be evaluated as well as the environmental conditions of the room.

---

environmental enrichment

The controlled environment of the research guinea pigs may not provide adequate opportunity for social interaction and species typical behaviors. To better provide for these needs, one or more of the following may be added to the husbandry practices:

1. Guinea pigs are social creatures and do very well in group housing situations. Animals may be housed as a pair (one male and one female), in polygamous groups (one male with numerous females), or in same sex groups.[89] Not all animals will adjust and tolerate this housing system. Aggression between guinea pigs may occur, but is usually not severe.

2. Interactions with animal care personnel, such as handling and petting, may provide adequate stimuli for the guinea pig.

3. Introduction of novel food items may allow guinea pigs to forage and gnaw. These may include grains, wooden chew sticks, and fresh fruits or vegetables. However, due to the fastidious nature of guinea pigs, these items may not be accepted by some animals.

> **Note:** When using fresh fruits or vegetables in the diet, care must be taken not to inadvertently introduce bacteria, such as Salmonella and Listeria, or other pathogens into the guinea pig's environment.

4. Introduction of novel items or "toys" into the cage. These include such things as chew toys, balls, paper tubes, and sections of plastic pipe. All items should be easy to sanitize and free of sharp edges.

5. Sensory enrichment with a softly playing radio may be beneficial to easily frightened species such as the guinea pig. This should provide a *soft* background noise to mask louder noises.[94]

6. Providing bedding and nesting materials is also beneficial to guinea pigs. Bedding should be provided in solid bottom cages, while nesting materials may also be provided for pregnant and nonpregnant animals. Choices of bedding materials have been previously discussed. Nesting materials can include paper towels or commercially available "nestlets". however, pregnant guinea pigs rarely build a true nest for the young.

> **Note:** When attempting to enrich the environment of guinea pigs, it must be remembered that these are creatures of habit and familiarity and may not always tolerate novel changes in their environment.

nutrition

Guinea pigs are strict herbivores with a unique requirement for vitamin C not seen in other rodents. They are fastidious eaters that begin to discriminate between edible and non-edible items within a few days of birth.[95] They are also messy eaters, dropping and wasting a good portion of their feed.

The following points should be considered with respect to feed:

1. The amount of feed given to guinea pigs should be unlimited or *ad libitum*. However, this may vary according to the age, sex, and research protocol. Guinea pigs do not adjust well to limited feeding.[95] Commercially available guinea pig feed is a plant based pelleted diet, that resembles rabbit food, that provides total nutrition.

2. Presentation of feed is usually via a J-feeder attached to the outside of the cage. Guinea pigs are known for using feed bowls placed on the cage floor as nests or toilets, which makes the use of these feeders less than desirable. Introduction of a new diet should be done by mixing the new diet with the old diet in increasing quantities until a complete transition has been made. Powdered foods may need to be moistened to a doughy consistency before they are accepted. These methods will prevent the accidental starvation of animals that may occur when guinea pigs are presented with unfamiliar food and refuse to eat.

3. Guinea pigs have a high requirement for various amino acids. This is met by providing a diet of 20% plant origin protein.[89] Alfalfa is a common source of this protein.

4. An adequate amount of fiber is necessary for optimal digestive tract function in guinea pigs. This requirement is also frequently met with dietary alfalfa and represents 10 to 18% of the diet.[95]

5. Vitamin C (ascorbic acid) is a daily requirement in the diet of guinea pigs. It is heat sensitive and easily oxidized. Guinea pigs, along with humans and nonhuman primates, lack one of the enzymes needed to convert glucose to ascorbic acid. Commercial guinea pig feed contains

adequate quantities of this vitamin under normal storage and use conditions. If the diet must be autoclaved, it should be a diet with additional quantities of vitamin C. A deficiency of vitamin C produces scurvy, with clinical signs of reluctance to move (pain) and anorexia and necropsy evidence of hemorrhage, opportunistic infections, and bony change. Experimental diets that lack adequate vitamin C may be supplemented by giving the animals ascorbic acid (25 to 50 mg/day) by gavage.[95,96] A complete discussion of this nutritional disease may be found in Chapter 4.

6. Vitamin E deficiency in guinea pigs has been associated with skeletal muscle degeneration, fetal malformation and resorption, paralysis, and testicular degeneration. A daily replacement dosage of 15 mg may be necessary to regain whole body vitamin E levels.[89,95]

7. Vitamin A deficiency and excess in guinea pigs have been associated with poor growth and eye abnormalities (deficiency) and fetal malformation (excess). A replacement of dosage of 1.5mg/day is sufficient to restore normal levels.[95]

8. Vitamin D deficiency, or an imbalance of calcium and phosphorus, can lead to rickets in guinea pigs with clinical signs of broadened cartilage plates and hypoplasia of incisors. If calcium and phosphorus balance is appropriate, guinea pigs can tolerate vitamin D deficiency without producing clinical signs.[95]

9. An appropriate balance of calcium, phosphorus, magnesium, potassium, and hydrogen ions is necessary for the good health of guinea pigs. These nutrients regulate acid-base balance and blood pH. An inappropriate balance of these nutrients has also been associated with metastatic calcification, along with vitamin D, leading to muscle stiffness and kidney malfunction.[95]

10. Storage of feed from commercial sources should be in a temperature controlled (50°F) room, without excess humidity. It should be stored away from pesticides, cleaning chemicals, and other items that would be harmful to the guinea pigs if ingested. Extra feed, except for

the bag currently being used, should not be stored in the animal room. Guinea pig feed will maintain adequate nutritive value for 90 days from the milling date. This is due to the lability of vitamin C. The milling date may be found on the outside of the bag of feed as a readable date or a code. Ask the vendor for a key to this code.

The open bag of feed currently being used should be stored in a vermin proof container with a sealable lid. This may then be kept within the animal room. When this bag is first opened, the milling date (or expiration date) should be recorded on the sealable container using white tape or in a record book.

11. Guinea pigs are coprophagic. They eat fecal pellets directly from the anus or, if they are obese or pregnant, from the cage floor. This activity appears to be necessary for optimal health and may increase the guinea pigs intake of protein, B vitamins, and fiber. Young guinea pigs consume the mother's fecal pellets to inoculate their intestinal tract with the proper microbes necessary for good digestion.[89]

12. Water should be provided *ad libitum*. It should be clean, fresh, and free of contaminants. Guinea pigs consume 100 mL/kg/day. The water may be provided in water bottles, crocks, or automatic watering devices. Guinea pigs enjoy playing in their water and may inadvertently flood their own cage or contaminate the water bottle or crock by putting feed or bedding into the water. Fresh drinking water should be provided daily.

Note: Rabbit food should never be fed to guinea pigs. Rabbit food lacks vitamin C and will produce scurvy in guinea pigs.

---

sanitation

A good animal care program involves the intertwined workings of housing, nutrition, environmental enrichment, healthy animals, and animal care personnel and practices. Another major factor in this equation is proper sanitation practices. To accomplish this goal, items such as frequency of sanitation, methods of sanitation, and quality control to monitor effectiveness must be addressed.

Frequency of sanitation practices for cages and animal rooms is variable and depends upon a number of factors including the number of guinea pigs per cage, animal age, number of cages per room, caging system, type of feed, and research practices and procedures.

1. Daily sanitation practices should include removal of dirty and wet bedding from solid bottom cages or removal of urine and feces beneath suspended cages, monitoring and cleaning of automatic watering valves or replacing dirty water bottles, and sweeping or damp-mopping the floor of the animal room.

2. Weekly sanitation practices should include transfer of animals to clean, disinfected cages with a clean waterer and feeder, however, this may done every two weeks under appropriate conditions. Cleaning and sanitation of room equipment, such as sinks and countertops, complete replacement of bedding in solid bottom cages, disinfection of litter trays beneath suspended cages, if used, should also be done weekly. Any cage that is found to be wet or exceptionally dirty should be changed at that time.

3. Cage racks should be changed with clean, disinfected cage racks monthly.

4. The entire animal room should be cleaned and disinfected at the conclusion of the study or whenever the room is empty of animals. Complete sanitization of the room at least every six months is recommended. This may require moving existing animals to another clean, disinfected room.

Sanitation methods may vary between institutions but should generally adhere to the following. Methods for the disinfection of caging equipment should include:

1. Removal of grossly visible organic material such as hair, feed, bedding, feces, and urine scale, from the large volume of protein and mineral containing urine guinea pigs excrete.[88] This may be accomplished by brushing the surfaces and rinsing with water; however, the use of detergents may facilitate the procedure. Tenacious urine scale may require prewashing/soaking the cage or litter pan in dilute organic acid. Phosphoric acid or citric acid are frequently used. Individuals involved with these procedures should wear the appropriate protective clothing to prevent chemical and/or thermal burns. This should include protection of skin, eyes, and nasal passages.

2. Cage washers are the most frequently used means of cage and equipment cleaning and disinfection. They employ the use of detergents, disinfectants, and hot water. However, these same functions may be performed efficiently by hand, as documented with rabbit caging.[97] Whenever chemicals are used as part of the sanitization program, thorough rinsing of this equipment with water must occur. This prevents the accidental exposure of the animals and personnel to these products. Rinse water temperatures of 180°F for 15 minutes have been found to effectively disinfect cages and equipment, as have lower temperatures for longer periods of time.[98]

> **Note:** Personnel performing cleaning and sanitizing procedures should always wear protective equipment such as gloves, aprons, safety goggles and/or face shields, and respirators.

Disinfection of guinea pig rooms should include:

1. Removal of all gross debris by rinsing with water. Detergents and brushing may be necessary for removal of adherent debris followed by rinsing with clear water.

2. Disinfection of room surfaces is accomplished by the application of one of a various number of commercial chemicals. The amount of contact time required for the

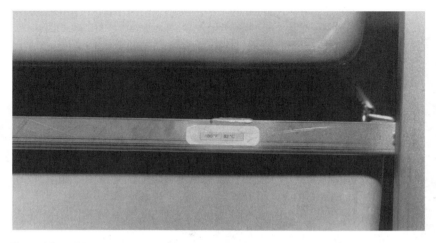

Fig. 18. Heat-sensitive temperature tape attached to a stainless steel cage rack before washing. This tape will turn dark when the appropriate temperature has been reached.

surface to be disinfected is dependent on the chemical used and manufacturer's recommendations. After adequate contact time, the surfaces should be thoroughly rinsed with clear water.

Note: Guinea pigs should never be left in the room during any room sanitation procedures.

All sanitation procedures should be monitored for effectiveness by a good quality control program. This program should be well documented and a written record maintained of all procedures. One or both of the following methods may be used to achieve this goal, however, use of both is recommended.

1. Heat-sensitive temperature tapes may be applied to equipment undergoing heat disinfection, such as with the use of cage washers (Figure 18). These tapes change color when the appropriate temperature has been reached. Used tapes should be dated and retained in a record book.

2. Microbiological monitoring involves the culture of bacteria and fungus still found on the surfaces of cages,

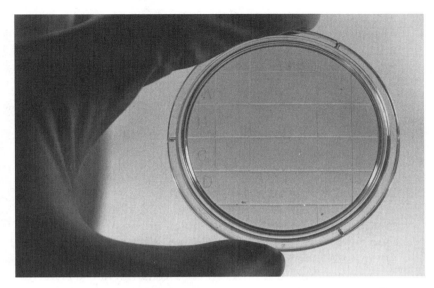

Fɪɢ. 19. Gridded RODAC plate to be used to monitor effectiveness of sanitation procedures. Plate is pressed against clean surfaces and cultured for bacterial and fungal contamination.

equipment, rooms, water bottles, sipper tubes, and feeders after sanitization procedures have been completed. This is done by swabbing the area of interest and culturing or by applying RODAC plates directly to the surface of interest (Figure 19) and then incubating these plates. The cleanliness of the surface is then known by the number and type of bacteria and fungus grown. Records of the results of these procedures should also be maintained.

transportation

Infrequently guinea pigs will need to be transported between buildings, facilities, or institutions. Laws governing and recommendations for the transportation of guinea pigs may be found within the *Animal Welfare Act* and the *Guide for the Care and Use of Laboratory Animals* and are included below.[83,84] Factors to be considered include housing during transport, access to food and water, clinical observation of the guinea pigs, and environmental conditions.

1. The shipping container housing the guinea pig must be strong enough to withstand the rigors of shipping and securely contain the animals within. It should provide adequate ventilation without drafts and be free of sharp edges that could injure the guinea pigs. If a corrugated cardboard container is used, surfaces must be laminated or covered with wire mesh to prevent escape. Groups must be compatible and adequate space must be provided for each animal. Bedding or another means of waste containment should be provided.

2. Food and water must be provided if the transit time is greater than six hours. However, under more extreme environmental conditions it may be necessary to provide food and water for trips less than six hours in length. Quantities of food and water should be sufficient to meet the normal fluid and nutrient requirements of the guinea pigs within the container. Commercially prepared products designed to meet these requirements are available.

3. During transport, the guinea pigs must be observed at least every four hours. The well-being of the guinea pig, environmental conditions, and adequate ventilation should be monitored at these times. If an animal is found in ill health it should receive prompt veterinary care.

4. The environmental conditions surrounding the guinea pig are of great importance. Guinea pigs are very heat sensitive and easily succumb to heat stress/stroke. They tolerate cool temperatures better, but are also highly sensitive to drafts and cold.

record keeping

Record keeping with well maintained documentation provides proof of acceptable animal care and use standards. The basis of a good record keeping program relies on having all information needed in written form, that is easily understood and completed, and that is readily accessible to those needing the information. These documents should be kept for a designated period of time in a manner that protects them from destruction and theft. All

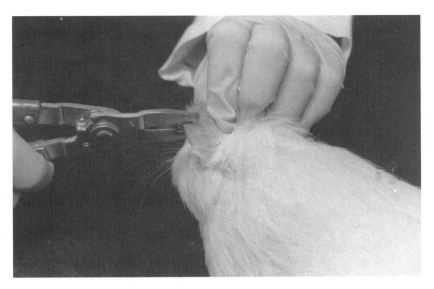

Fig. 20.   Proper placement of a metal, numbered ear tag in the ear of a guinea pig for individual identification.

personnel working with the guinea pigs should understand the necessity for and importance of these documents and be willing to follow procedures.

The backbone of proper record keeping is the identification of animals. Guinea pigs may be identified individually by ear tag (Figure 20), ear notch or punch (Figure 21), subcutaneous transponders, tattoo, or coloration of the fur, with permanent dyes or a marking pen (short term identification only). If all animals in a cage are being treated exactly the same, then the animals may be identified as a group by the use of a cage card. This card should contain the number of animals, species of animal, strain of animal, any distinct physical features, any identifying marks, sex of the animals, and research protocol and/or responsible investigator. For maintenance of a breeding colony or varied research parameters, individual identification is recommended.[83,88]

Basic records that should be maintained by the research facility include, but are not limited to, the following:

1.   Health records should be maintained on every guinea pig, or group as identified above. This should include the general health of the animal, such as activity level, alertness,

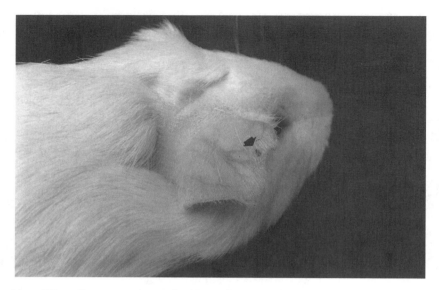

FIG. 21.   Guinea pig with a single, circular ear punch for individual identification.

appetite, urination and defecation, and any abnormalities. Documentation of experimental manipulations and veterinary treatments should also be included.

2.   An accurate census of the number of animals in each room and within the facility is necessary for the assignment of daily tasks to animal care personnel and the appropriate assignment of housing per diem rates.

3.   Work records recording routine husbandry tasks should also be maintained. These should include, usually in a check off format, provision of food and water, cage cleaning, changing of cages and racks, room temperature, date that specific procedures were performed, and initials of person performing tasks.

management

The management of a facility housing guinea pigs is governed by numerous governmental agencies and regulatory bodies. These include local and state agencies, which may have varying regulations and requirements between locations. The federal government in the United States has three primary organizations that regulate, oversee, and accredit the use of guinea pigs in research, teaching, and testing.

regulatory agencies and compliance

The United States Department of Agriculture (USDA)

- The Animal and Plant Health Inspection Service (APHIS) of USDA has oversight and enforcement responsibility for the use of guinea pigs as described in the Animal Welfare Act (AWA) and its amendments (P.L. 91-579, P.L. 94-279, P.L. 99-198).[99]

- The specific requirements of the AWA are found within the Regulations of the Animal Welfare Act document.[84]

- These regulations require all facilities using guinea pigs for research, teaching, and testing, except elementary and secondary schools, to register with USDA and adhere to these regulations.

The National Institutes of Health (NIH), Public Health Service (PHS)

- The Health Extension Act of 1985 (P.L 99-158) designates oversight responsibility of this act to the Director of NIH. The Office for Protection from Research Risks (OPRR) is the coordination and administration agency for these regulations.[100]

- The Public Health Service Policy on Humane Care and Use of Laboratory Animals describes the contents of this act.[101]

- Recommendations for the implementation of this act and its policy are found in the *Guide for the Care and Use of Laboratory Animals* (frequently referred to as the *Guide*).[83]

- This policy must be followed by any institution receiving funds from PHS.

- Every institution must file with OPRR an Animal Welfare Assurance document, detailing program policies.

The United States Food and Drug Administration (FDA) and the Environmental Protection Agency (EPA).

- The Good Laboratory Practices for Nonclinical Laboratory Studies document describes the procedures and policies of these agencies.[102]

- These regulations must be followed when guinea pigs are used in studies to seek approval or marketing permits for drugs and medical devices intended for human use (FDA) or herbicides and fungicides (EPA).

- Copious recordkeeping involving standard operating procedures, data collection, and quality control are the basis of these regulations.

Association for Assessment and Accreditation of Laboratory Animal Care International, Inc. (AAALAC International)

- AAALAC International is a nonprofit, accrediting body designed to identify and monitor institutions that use animals for research, teaching, or testing that meet or exceed the standards set forth in the *Guide for the Care and Use of Laboratory Animals.*[83]

- Participation is voluntary.

- Accreditation involves site visits, program reviews, and triennial revisits by selected peers.

institutional animal care and use committee (iacuc)

The oversight and internal management of the care and use of guinea pigs used in research, teaching, and testing lies with the IACUC. This committee and its powers and responsibilities are described in the Guide, the Animal Welfare Act, and the PHS Policy.[83,84,101] Therefore, this committee is also required for AAA-LAC accreditation. The following delineate some of the points relevant to the IACUC in these documents.

1. The minimum number of members on the committee must be three, as described by USDA, however, the PHS policy requires a minimum of five persons. These persons are to be appointed by the chief executive officer of the institution.

2. The qualification of the members of the committee must include the following (the first three by USDA and all five by PHS):

    - A chairperson.

    - A Doctor of Veterinary Medicine with training or experience in laboratory animal science and medicine who has responsibility for the activities involving research animals.

    - A person not affiliated with the institution in any way or any other IACUC member. Some examples of acceptable persons include lawyers, clergy, or animal shelter or humane society officials.

    - A practicing scientist with experience in animal research.

- A person whose primary concerns are in a nonscientific area. This person may be employed by the institution.

- The PHS policy states that one person may fulfill more than one of the above requirements, however, the committee must still contain the minimum number of persons (5).

- The USDA requires that no more than three members of the committee shall be from the same administrative unit, however, the committee must have more than three members.

3. The responsibilities of the IACUC are delineated in the current regulations, which should be consulted for specifics, and include the following:

- Review the facility's program for humane care and use of animals at least once every six months.

- Inspect all animal facilities at least once every six months and assure that they are appropriate for the species housed within.

- Prepare reports describing the results of the above evaluations and submit these to the Institutional Official. The Institutional Official is the person at a facility who is authorized to legally commit on behalf of the facility. This position is frequently filled by a Vice President.

- Review proposed protocols for the use of guinea pigs in research. An approved protocol must be in place before animal use can begin. Significant changes to the approved protocols must also be approved before they may be implemented.

- Assure that appropriate sedation, anesthesia, analgesia, and euthanasia methods are used so that there is minimal discomfort, distress, and pain.

- Assure that appropriate surgical and recovery methods are used.

- Assure that the principal investigator (PI) has considered alternatives to procedures that may cause more than momentary or slight pain or distress.

- Obtain written assurance from the PI that the proposed research does not unnecessarily duplicate previous experiments.

- Assure that all persons performing procedures on animals are qualified and properly trained in those procedures.

---

occupational health and zoonotic diseases

The Animal Welfare Act and PHS Policy both require an occupational health and safety program be in place for personnel working with regulated research animals.[84,101] The *Guide* also makes recommendations for this program.[83] However, Bowman has described a comprehensive occupational health and safety program which could be used, sometimes with modifications, under most circumstances.[103] In the development or adaptation of an occupational health and safety program for personnel using guinea pigs, the following aspects need to be considered:

1. The purchase of purpose bred guinea pigs will greatly reduce the chances of encountering a zoonotic disease agent, however, a few bacteria carried by guinea pigs have the potential to infect humans even though few cases have been documented. Under research conditions, it may be just as likely that these agents are transmitted from human hosts to the guinea pig. A more thorough discussion of some of these agents may be found in the following chapter.

   - *Streptococcus pneumoniae* may cause respiratory and meningeal disease in humans.

   - Other Streptococci may infect skin wounds.

   - *Salmonella spp.* are known to cause mild to severe gastrointestinal disease in people.

- Dermatophytes (ringworm), usually asymptomatic in the guinea pig, may produce circular, pruritic skin lesions in humans.

- *Chlamydia psittaci* is known to produce respiratory disease in people, however, no cases have been attributed to guinea pigs.

- Cryptosporidium sp. are not species specific, but are believed to be separate species with different host ranges and are known to produce intestinal disease in humans and guinea pigs.

- *Trixacarus caviae* can cause pruritic skin lesions in people.

2. Skin wounds are a very common problem in the animal care facility. They may be the result of the occasional guinea pig bite or toenail scratch. However, puncture wounds and lacerations from sharp edges or protrusions on metal equipment are far more frequent. Therefore, a current tetanus vaccination is recommended for anyone working in the facility.

3. Allergies to guinea pigs are also common. Allergic reactions may vary from mild respiratory signs; such as sneezing, rhinitis, and pruritic eyes; and skin symptoms; such as erythema, pruritus, and edema; to severe clinical disease; such as anaphylaxis or asthma. Sensitive individuals should cover exposed skin and mucous membranes when working with the guinea pigs or in the guinea pig room. Appropriate protective equipment would include a clean labcoat or coveralls, gloves, and a face mask or respirator. Equipment should be laundered or cleaned frequently. It is wise for less sensitive individuals to follow these same precautions because severe allergies can develop with continued exposure to the animal dander. The best solution to severe allergic reactions is to avoid exposure to the allergen. This usually involves reassignment of sensitive personnel or a change in research species of interest and consultation with an expert in the field of occupational health and safety.

4. Many research projects involve the use of infectious agents. These experimental biohazards require the use of set procedures for handling the infected animals, animals wastes, animal tissues, and housing equipment. Specific recommendations for these procedures have been published by the Centers for Disease Control (CDC).[104]

5. The use of many toxic chemicals for cleaning and experimentation pose another potential hazard. Set protocols and personal protective equipment should also be implemented in these situations A hazardous materials specialist should be consulted for specifics.

6. The use of washable labcoats or coveralls and gloves, along with frequent hand washing and a cautious attitude, represent the basis for protection from most research hazards. The addition of specific personal protective equipment when appropriate, such as goggles, face shields, and respirators, and their proper use, should provide protection for anyone using laboratory guinea pigs in research, teaching, or testing.

animal health monitoring program

Guinea pigs used for research should be obtained from a reputable vendor and known to be free of disease. However, animals that are maintained within the facility for more than six months or a room of animals that are maintained for more than six months with animals going in and out of the room without complete emptying of the room should be involved in a health monitoring program. This program should monitor for the accidental introduction of disease into the colony or room. Each individual program will vary based upon the number of guinea pigs maintained, other species in facility, intensity of program, and finances. The *Guide* recommends such a program.[83] A good health monitoring program is described elsewhere.[105,106] The design and implementation of a health monitoring program should consider the following:

- Serology for antibodies to microorganisms is the most important part. Some programs may only include this procedure. Sendai virus, pneumonia virus of mice, *Clostridium piliforme*, lymphocytic choriomeningitis virus, cytomegalovirus, reovirus type 3, simian virus 5, and *Encepalitozoon cuniculi* are diseases which may be monitored.

- Serology may be done with blood samples obtained without euthanizing the guinea pigs.

- Monitoring may be done one, two or four time a year, however, two or more is recommended.

- A complete program includes not only serology, but also necropsy, histopathology, bacterial culture, and parasite evaluation.

- The number of animals evaluated may vary, but usually requires a minimum of four to five animals.

- Serologic monitoring of animals recently received from a vendor is recommended to verify their health status.

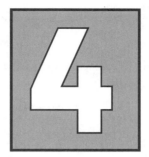

veterinary care

basic veterinary supplies

A few recommended supplies and equipment should be maintained for basic veterinary care of guinea pigs. This could include the following, however, additional items may be needed for varying animal care protocols:

- A stethoscope.

- A small animal rectal thermometer.

- Tube of lubricant.

- Nail clippers.

- An assortment of disposable hypodermic needles varying in size from 21 to 26 gauge (diameter) and 5/8 to 1 1/2 inches long.

- An assortment of syringes varying in size from 1 mL to 12 mL.

- Blood collection tubes without additives (or with coagulation accelerator, for serum) or with added sodium EDTA (for whole blood).

- Sterile fluids such as lactated Ringer's solution, 0.9% saline, and/or 5% glucose.

- Swabs with transport media for bacterial culture.

- Gauze sponges.

- Skin disinfectant scrub or solution such as providone-iodine or chlorhexidine.

- Stainless steel feeding tube, 16 gauge, 4 inches long, for oral dosing.

- Urine dipstick for ketone bodies (if breeding females are maintained).

physical examination of the guinea pig

Newly received guinea pigs should be examined prior to introduction into a facility, and at any other time that abnormalities are noted. A thorough physical examination should be methodical, systematically covering all portions of the animal's body. Results of these examinations should be maintained in the animal's medical record.

- Begin the examination with a general assessment of the animal's overall appearance and behavior. Note if activity and strength appear normal. Observe the gait and balance as the animal moves about the cage, and behavior during removal from the cage.

- Observe the feces and urine in the cage pan or bedding. The amount, color, and consistency of the feces and urine should be noted.

- The food bowl and water bottle (if used) should be checked to see if appetite and water intake are normal.

- Examine the coat for smoothness, cleanliness, hair loss, skin lesions, and skin masses. A normal guinea pig should have a smooth, full, well-groomed haircoat.

- Examine the feet and nails for sores, and torn or broken nails.

- Palpate all four limbs.

- Examine the eyes for discharge or reddening of the conjunctiva.

- The nose should also be examined for discharge.

- Look at the mouth and lips, with close inspection of the teeth and oral cavity. The small size of the mouth opening can make this difficult, but use of a mouth speculum and a penlight aid the process. A disposable syringe case or barrel of a syringe can be used as a makeshift speculum.

- Examine the ears for inflammation or discharge and submandibular area for swellings.

- Auscultate the thorax with a stethoscope. This is difficult but may provide useful information about the presence or absence of abnormal respiratory sounds.

- Observe the rate and character of respirations.

- Palpate the abdomen for masses. This procedure is best performed by holding the guinea pig on its back, and palpating with the opposite hand. Systematically palpate in a cranial to caudal direction.

- Examine the perineum for urine or fecal staining, discharges, or other abnormalities.

- The animal's temperature may be taken rectally using a well-lubricated small animal thermometer. A digital thermometer with a smaller, more tapered probe or an infrared tympanic thermometer may be easier to use, although the accuracy of this method has not been established for the guinea pig.

quarantine

New guinea pigs that have just arrived at the facility should be maintained in housing separated from all other animals. This may be a separate room, cubicle, or ventilated rack. They should remain in quarantine for one to two weeks. If no health problems are encountered, then they may be moved into rooms or areas containing other animals. The positive effects of this quarantine and conditioning period are well documented.[107]

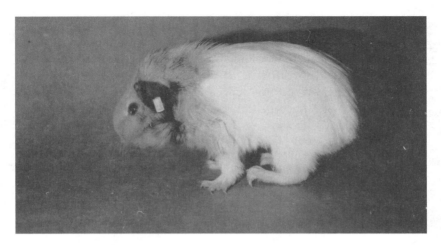

Fig. 22. Clinically ill guinea pig demonstrating hunched posture: "tucked-up" abdomen, scruffy coat, weight loss, and general ill appearance.

clinical signs of illness in guinea pigs

- A sick guinea pig will commonly have a reduced appetite and weight loss. Moderate to severe weight loss can be observed as a drawing in of the flanks, and loss of the rounded contour of the abdomen (Figure 22).

- Hair may stick up, giving the animal a rough, unkempt appearance.

- The animal may appear lethargic and disinterested in its surroundings.

- Ocular or nasal discharge, or diarrhea may be present.

common clinical problems

Summarized here are a number of the more common clinical diseases found in guinea pigs, with a brief discussion of etiology, presentation, diagnostic procedure, and control or treatment recommendations. Clinical presentations and specific etiologies are found in Table 8.

TABLE 8.   COMMON DISEASES OF GUINEA PIGS

Clinical signs/disease	Etiology
Pneumonia	*Bordetella bronchiseptica, Streptococcus pneumoniae*
Conjuctivitis	*Chlamydia psittaci, Bordetella bronchiseptica, Streptococcus pneumoniae*
Diarrhea	*Clostridium piliforme,* cryptosporidiosis, protozoan (other), antibiotic toxicity
Weight loss	Malocclusion, nutritional deficiency, cryptosporidiosis, systemic disease
Acute death	Salmonellosis, campylobacteriosis, typhlocolitis, antibiotic toxicity, pregnancy toxemia, dystocia, dehydration, hyperthermia, hypothermia
Abortion	Salmonellosis, pregnancy toxemia, cytomegalovirus, nutritional deficiency
Masses/swellings	Cervical lymphadenitis (*S. zooepidemicus*), tumor, scurvy (joints), mastitis
Alopecia	Barbering, gestational alopecia, external parasites
Lameness	Scurvy, pododermatitis
Neurologic disease (torticollis)	Lymphocytic choriomeningitis, toxoplasmosis, *S. pneumoniae, B. bronchiseptica*

> **Note:**   Guinea pigs are prone to a number of health problems. Many of these may be avoided with good husbandry and sanitation practices, and by careful selection of animals from reputable vendors. If health problems are suspected a veterinarian with expertise with guinea pigs should be consulted.

Vitamin C Deficiency (Scurvy)

- Guinea pigs, like primates (including man), have a genetic absence of l-gulonolactone oxidase, an enzyme critical for the formation of ascorbic acid.

- Storage of vitamin C in tissues is poor in the guinea pig, and is insufficient for periods of inadequate intake. Daily intake of vitamin C in a high-quality food or a dietary supplement is necessary to prevent scorbutism (scurvy).

- Scurvy, particularly subclinical cases, may be more common than is generally recognized.[108]

- Clinically, animals have a rough haircoat, diarrhea, reluctance to move, and anorexia.

- Collagen synthesis defects and impaired clotting mechanisms result in delayed healing, joint swelling and lameness, and hemorrhages in multiple tissues.[109]

- Diagnosis is based on observation of the clinical signs, investigation of the diet, and necropsy of affected individuals.

- Necropsy findings include enlargement of the costochondral junctions of the ribs, and muscle and subcutaneous hemorrhages as seen in Figure 23.

- Treatment of affected individuals consists of immediate supplementation with vitamin C (10 mg/kg parenterally, daily, for at least one week), correction of the diet, and supportive care (fluid therapy, supplemental feeding). Kale, cabbage, and citrus fruits are excellent supplemental sources of vitamin C.

- If drinking water is supplemented (200mg/L), the vitamin C solution is unstable and must be changed daily.

- Pelleted guinea pig feeds must be properly stored under dry conditions, protected from heat and sunlight, and must be used within 90 days of the milling date.

Bordetella bronchiseptica

- Guinea pigs are uniquely susceptible to infection with *Bordetella bronchiseptica*, a Gram-negative, non-spore forming rod.

- *Bordetella* is harbored by numerous species including man and rabbits and is easily spread by aerosols and contaminated fomites.

- Young and stressed guinea pigs are most at risk for infection.

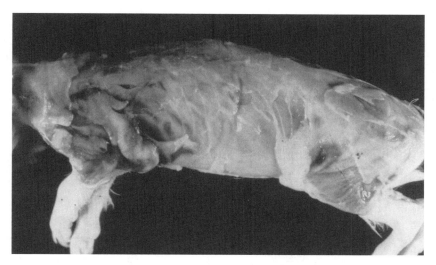

FIG. 23. Body of a scorbutic, hypovitaminosis C, guinea pig with subcutaneous, muscular, and joint hemorrhages.

- Asymptomatic carriers harbor the organism in the nasal cavity and trachea.

- Infected animals may exhibit dyspnea, nasal discharge, loss of appetite, or depression, but often they are found dead without obvious antemortem signs.

- Necropsy may reveal blood tinged fluid in the trachea, consolidated lungs (Figure 24), tracheitis, bronchopneumonia, and infection in the middle ear.

- Diagnosis is based on necropsy findings and confirmed by culture and isolation of the organism.

- Prevention of the disease is preferred to treatment, with attention to vendor selection and routine health monitoring of the colony.

- Vaccination with a killed bacterin has been shown to protect animals for several months; repeated use of a bacterin can eliminate the organism from a colony.[110,111]

- Chloramphenicol and sulfa-based antibiotics may be helpful in treating sick animals.

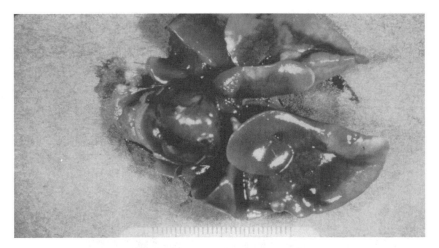

FIG. 24. Consolidated, pneumonic lungs taken from a guinea pig with *Bordetella bronchiseptica* pneumonia. (Courtesy of Dr. Joseph E. Wagner.)

Streptococcus pneumoniae

- This Gram-positive coccus bacteria is usually found arranged in pairs or chains.

- It may be carried in the respiratory passages of apparently normal guinea pigs, as well as being carried by numerous other species including humans.

- Active disease is more commonly found in stressed animals, where poor husbandry, shipping, pregnancy, temperature changes, or experimental protocols are a factor.

- Affected animals are inactive, have a rough hair coat, and a poor appetite.

- Nasal discharge and dyspnea may be observed; pregnant sows may abort.

- Death is often the only sign noted.

- Diagnosis is based on clinical signs, necropsy findings, and isolation of the organism.

- Postmortem findings include edematous lungs, purulent processes affecting a number of organs: pleuritis, pericarditis, abscesses in the lungs, otitis, and others.[112,113]

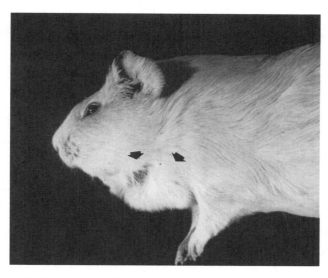

Fig. 25. Guinea pig with large ventral cervical swellings with typical lymphadenitis.

- Treatment with antibiotics may control an epidemic, but does not eliminate the carriers in the colony.[114]

- Prevention by maintaining a closed colony, vendor selection, and good husbandry practices are the preferred methods of control.

Cervical Lymphadenitis

- Animals present with lumpy swellings under the chin which are enlarged submandibular lymph nodes (Figure 25). Usually, no other clinical signs are observed. Lymph nodes in other areas of the body are infrequently involved. Occasionally an animal may become systemically ill, developing pneumonia, otitis, or sepsis.

- Swollen lymph nodes contain abscesses filled with a thick, yellow, purulent material. *Streptococcus zooepidemicus*, a Gram-positive cocci, can be isolated from the draining material.[112]

- The condition is treated by draining the abscess or allowing them to rupture and drain spontaneously.

- The method of transmission is not well understood, but culling infected animals from the colony may reduce the spread of the organism. It has been suggested, and refuted, that the organism gains entry through abraded oral mucosa, and is spread by carrier animals.[115]

Antibiotic Toxicity

- Guinea pigs normally have a primarily Gram-positive enteric flora. Antibiotics, particularly those with a spectrum targeting the Gram-positive organisms, can cause an alteration to Gram-negative microbes resulting in acute enterocolitis, sepsis or toxemia, and death.[116-118]

- Animals are often found dead following antibiotic administration with no previous clinical signs.

- Those that do not die acutely may exhibit anorexia, dehydration, and hypothermia before death.

- There is no treatment, but avoiding antibiotic usage effectively prevents the condition. Penicillins, lincomycin, clindamycin, erythromycin, chlortetracycline, oxytetracycline, bacitracin, and streptomycin have all been implicated.[116]

> **Note:** Broad spectrum antibiotics such as chloramphenicol and enrofloxacin are relatively less risky, but when giving antibiotics to a guinea pig carefully weigh benefits vs. risks.

- A similar syndrome occurs in guinea pigs with no history of antibiotic exposure, where apparently healthy animals are suddenly found dead.

- Necropsy findings include necrosis and inflammation of the cecal and intestinal mucosa. Cases are sometimes associated with steroid administration, pregnancy, and experimental protocols that change the bacterial flora of the intestines or otherwise stress the guinea pig.

- The phenomenon suggests the cause is an enteric bacterial flora disturbance similar to that found in antibiotic toxicity.[112]

Pregnancy Toxemia

- Like human females, guinea pig females are susceptible to toxemia syndromes of pregnancy. This disorder in the guinea pig is a multifactorial metabolic disease with age, diet, obesity, fasting, exercise, fetal load, and heredity being contributing factors. Although most often associated with pregnancy, a similar metabolic disease (ketosis) is found occasionally in males and nonpregnant females.[119]

- Rapid mobilization of fat and increased production of ketones leading to ketonemia is the apparent mechanism.[120]

- Pregnant sows in their first or second gestation are most commonly affected. Most cases occur in late gestation, within 7 to 10 days of parturition.[121]

- Affected pigs become quiet, stop eating and drinking, have a ruffled haircoat, and lose weight. Eventually they become prostrate and die, usually within 2 to 4 days.

- Diagnosis is based on these clinical signs in obese or pregnant animals, a urine pH of 5 to 6, ketonuria, and hypoglycemia.[122]

- At necropsy, fatty livers (Figure 26) and hemorrhages or necrosis in the placenta are found.

- Once animals have developed clinical signs, treatment is unrewarding.

- Prevention of pregnancy ketosis is a more successful approach. Avoiding stresses such as moves and dietary changes, avoiding obesity in breeding females via limiting food intake, and breeding animals at smaller body weights are recommended measures.

Salmonellosis

- A devastating disease of guinea pigs, salmonellosis may be found worldwide. Several serotypes of the bacteria are known to have caused disease in animal colonies,

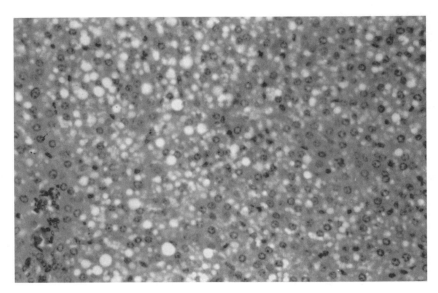

Fig. 26. Photomicrograph of a section of hematoxylin and eosin stained liver containing numerous fatty vacuoles. This is a frequent finding in guinea pigs with pregnancy toxemia.

including *Salmonella typhimurium*, *Salmonella enteriditis*, and *Salmonella dublin*.[112,123]

- Organisms are Gram-negative, non-spore forming, facultatively anaerobic bacilli.

- Infected animals rarely have diarrhea. Instead, a loss of appetite, rough haircut, weakness, and abortion in pregnant females may be found.

- All ages are affected, although young and stressed animals are the more severely affected.

- Mortality may exceed 50%.

- Recovered animals and asymptomatic carriers may spread the infection by intermittently shedding the organism in feces.

- Contamination of feed materials with the feces of wild rodents, especially fresh feeds such as cabbage or kale, may be a source of infection.

- At necropsy animals are found to have large spleens and lymph nodes, and whitish-colored nodules in the spleen, liver, and other organs.

- The diagnosis is confirmed with isolation of the organism from blood or swabs from the spleen.

- Treatment is not recommended, as recovered animals may be carriers of the organism. Destruction of the colony, with subsequent sanitation and restocking with clean animals appears to be the only course of action. Uninfected colonies can be protected by strict attention to sanitation, foregoing fresh greens in favor of a complete pelleted diet, and limiting or screening the admission of new animals.

> **Note:** Salmonella infections are zoonotic and may cause potentially serious disease in humans.

Alopecia

- Hair loss in guinea pigs has a number of different causes, with distinct patterns and presentations

- Barbering, or hair chewing may be the result of a dominance interaction between two guinea pigs or a behavioral vice. Animals may barber each other in a group housing situation, or may chew at their own hair. Typically, the hair loss is patchy with uneven hair lengths while the skin remains healthy and unabraded. Even though this condition is of no clinical significance, long stem hay may be provided to reduce the incidence.

- Gestational alopecia occurs in intensively bred females. Hair loss is a generalized thinning of the hair over the entire body (Figure 27). The presumed etiology is the hormonal influence of pregnancy, and reduced anabolism in maternal skin. Weanling guinea pigs have a similar alopecia for a short time when the "baby fur" is being replaced with a more adult, course fur.

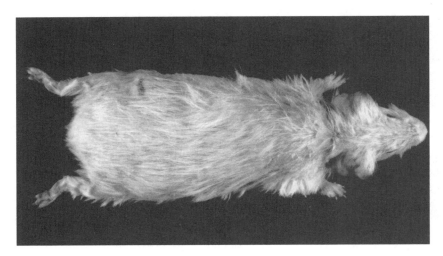

Fig. 27. Generalized alopecia in an adult female guinea pig. This condition is associated with intensive breeding and thought to be hormonal in etiology.

- Fungal Infections of the skin are common in guinea pigs. Infections may appear as patchy alopecia that spreads from the nose to other areas of the head, and eventually to the trunk. Limbs are often spared. Lesions usually involve the skin, producing scaly centers and redness along the borders. The characteristic circular lesion associated with "ringworm" may be seen (Figure 28), but should not be relied on for a diagnosis. Wood's lamp examination, fungal culture on Sabouraud's agar, and microscopic examination of potassium hydroxide prepared specimens confirm the diagnosis and identify the causative agent, usually *Microsporum canis* or *Trichophyton mentagrophytes*. For a potassium hydroxide preparation, a clump of hair collected from the edge of a lesion is placed in a few drops of potassium hydroxide on a slide and then examined under a microscope for indentification of fungal hyphae and conidia. Effective treatment of affected animals with griseofulvin, an orally administered antibiotic, has been reported.[124]

- External parasites, now relatively uncommon in laboratory guinea pigs, have been associated with hair loss.

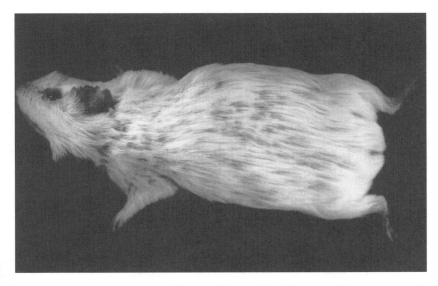

FIG. 28. Guinea pig with small circular lesions that are scaly in the center and erythematous around the edges. These lesions are frequently seen with dermatophyte ("ringworm") infections. (Courtesy of Dr. Joseph E. Wagner.)

Note: Fungal skin infections are zoonotic.

These pests are still found, mostly in pet or hobby colonies.

- *Chirodiscoides caviae,* a fur mite (Figure 29), can cause itching and hair loss if the infestation is heavy. There are no associated skin lesions. The mite can be identified by microscopic examination of the pelt, and is most easily found postmortem after the carcass has cooled. Frequently at necropsy, the pelt, or the portion of the pelt over the head, neck, and shoulders, is placed in a petri dish and allowed to cool. Then the dish is set on top of white paper and the pelt examined with a dissecting microscope. Mites can also be seen with the naked eye as small, dark, moving dots on the hair shaft.

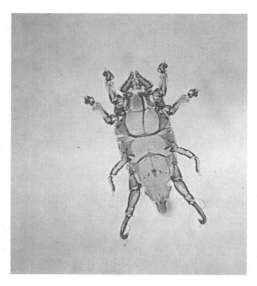

FIG. 29.   *Chirodiscoides caviae*, a guinea pig fur mite that may produce alopecia and itching in heavy infestations. (Courtesy of Dr. Joseph E. Wagner.)

- Another mite, *Trixacarus caviae* (Figure 30), burrows into the skin of guinea pigs, causing intense pruritus, alopecia, and thickening of the skin. Microscopic examination of skin scrapings are the preferred diagnostic tool.[125]

- Two species of lice have been associated with guinea pigs. *Gliricola porcelli* (Figure 31) and *Gyropus ovalis* are large, elongated arthropods. Both species are usually benign, but in heavy infestations can cause scratching, skin scabbing, and hair loss usually around the head and ears. Examination of the fur with a dissecting microscope or hand lens will usually detect the organisms.

- Treatment of external parasites consists of pyrethrin or carbaryl powders and dips, insecticide sprays, intensive room cleaning, ivermectin, and other reported agents.

Note: *Trixacarus caviae* has been reported to cause dermatitis in humans.

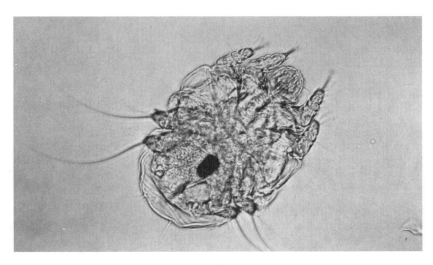

Fig. 30. *Trixacarus caviae*, a fur mite that burrows into the skin causing intense pruritis, alopecia, and skin changes. This mite also causes pruritis in humans. (Courtesy of Dr. Joseph E. Wagner.)

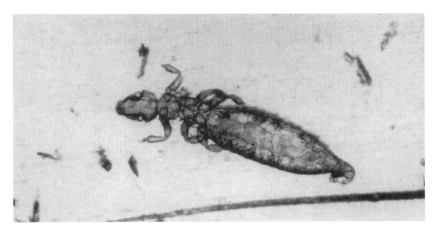

Fig. 31. *Gliricola porcelli*, one of the species of lice found in guinea pigs that may be associated with itching and hair loss. (Courtesy of Dr. Joseph E. Wagner.)

Malocclusion

- Continuous tooth growth throughout life, combined with dietary and genetic factors can result in uneven tooth wear and malocclusion in guinea pigs.[126,127]

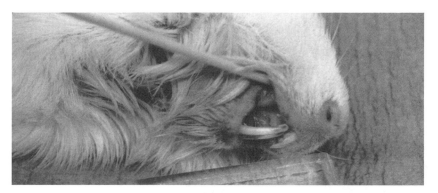

FIG. 32.   Overgrown incisors in a guinea pig secondary to overgrown premolars and molars producing malocclusion. (Courtesy of Dr. Joseph E. Wagner.)

- Cheek teeth (the premolars and anterior molars) are more commonly affected (Figure 32).[128]

- Because of the difficulty in examining these teeth, the condition is often overlooked until the incisors overgrow or the animal has a significant weight loss.

- Chronic weight loss and/or hypersalivation (slobbers) are indications that a thorough oral examination is needed.

- Cutting or filing the affected teeth provides temporary relief, but must be repeated at regular intervals throughout the animal's life. Teeth are cut by grinding or cutting with a high speed rotary tool. Large, side-cutting nail trimmers may also be used to trim the teeth, however, care must be taken to not crack the tooth.

Protozoal Diseases

- Several protozoan are known to infect guinea pigs.

- *Cryptosporidium wrairi* and *Eimeria caviae* are the most common of several protozoans that affect the intestinal tract of guinea pigs.

- Clinical signs vary from chronic weight loss to diarrhea.

- Although both organisms are capable of producing enteritis, the disease caused by *Eimeria* tends to be the more severe.[129]

- Postmortem examination of animals provides information about the specific agent. *Cryptosporidium* infections will produce lesions of chronic enteritis in the distal ileum, while *Eimeria* affects the colon producing nodules, hyperemia, and edema in affected tissue. Both can be definitively diagnosed by examination of mucosal scrapings or histopathology.

- Sulfamethazine in the water has been reported to eliminate *Eimeria* infections, but most epidemics of either can be prevented or minimized with proper cage design and good hygiene.[130]

- *Encephalitozoon cuniculi* is a protozoan capable of causing neurologic disease in several species of laboratory animals including guinea pigs, rabbits, and mice.[131]

  - The mode of infection is thought to be via oocytes shed in the urine.

  - Infected animals develop lesions in the brain and the kidney, microscopic granulomas containing the organism.[132]

  - Most infections are asymptomatic, but the disease may interfere with research by complicating interpretations of data.

  - There is no treatment.

  - Establishing and maintaining colonies of *E. cuniculi* free animals is the preferred approach.

Viral Diseases

- Several cytomegalovirus isolates have been identified that affect humans, mice, guinea pigs, and other species. Guinea pig cytomegalovirus, like those of other mammals, is a species-specific herpesvirus that can persist in infected hosts for long periods of time.

  - The virus is widespread in infected colonies, and disease is usually subclinical.

  - The uncommon clinical presentations are swelling of the salivary glands, fetal deaths, and acute death.[133,134]

- Microscopic examination of tissues reveals eosino-philic inclusion bodies in the ductal epithelium of salivary glands.

- Because the disease is spread transplacentally, no preventative measures are recommended other than careful selection of animals.

- Lymphocytic choriomeningitis occurs as a natural disease in the guinea pig.

  - A member of the arena virus group, this agent is not host specific and is capable of causing disease in many mammalian species including man.

  - The natural host, the mouse, can in some cases become an asymptomatic, sero-negative carrier of the disease, but this type of latent infection has not been confirmed in the guinea pig.

  - Clinical lymphocytic choriomeningitis (LCM) in guinea pigs is characterized by symptoms of meningitis and rear limb paralysis.

  - Pneumonia, fatty liver, and enlarged spleens may be found in infected animals in addition to the hallmark lymphocytic infiltrate in the meninges.

  - Serologic screening of sentinel animals can detect the presence of the disease in a group.

  - The virus may be spread by aerosol, biting insects, or contamination with urine. It may also be spread through the use of contaminated biologicals, such as tumors, injected into the guinea pig.

  - There is no treatment or control other than serologic surveillance, elimination of wild rodents, and sanitation.

Note: Lymphocytic choriomeningitis is a zoonotic disease capable of causing severe illness in humans.

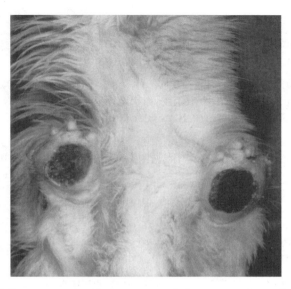

FIG. 33.   Ulceration and necrosis of the ventral surfaces of the front feet of a guinea pig. Pododermatitis ("bumblefoot") may affect one to all four feet. (Courtesy of Joseph E. Wagner.)

Pododermatitis

- Inflammation and sores on the footpads (Figure 33) are occasionally found in guinea pigs, causing lameness, stress, and failure to thrive.

- Dense body structure, obesity, wire-floored caging, and foot trauma contribute to the condition.

- Typically, this disease is associated with poor housing and poor sanitation.

- Once detected, the condition is treatable if not too far advanced. Affected animals should be placed on solid-floored housing, preferably on soft bedding. Housing should be kept as sanitary as possible with frequent bedding changes. Clipping hair from the lesions, cleaning the wounds, and the judicious use of topical antibiotics can speed the recovery of the animals.

Conjunctivitis

- Redness of eyelid margins and ocular discharge often indicate infection with *Chlamydia psittaci.*

- Usually seen in 1- to 3-week old animals, the disease is inapparent in many and spontaneously resolves in nearly all animals within 28 days of onset.

- Microscopic examination of conjunctival scrapings reveal intracytoplasmic inclusions within epithelial cells.[135]

- Since the disease is usually mild and self-limiting, there is no recommended treatment.

- This agent may provide a model for the study of trachoma, a similar, but often serious, human disease affecting millions worldwide.

- *Chlamydia psittaci* is potentially zoonotic.

general treatment of disease

Once a sick guinea pig has been identified, an appropriate diagnostic and treatment plan should be implemented under the direction of a qualified veterinarian. Listed in Table 9 are several drugs which may be used in guinea pigs, along with recommended dosages per unit of body weight. Abbreviations for frequency of administration are SID (once daily), BID (twice daily), and D (number of days). Routes of administration are abbreviated as PO (oral), IV (intravenous), IM (intramuscular), and SC (subcutaneous).

Small animals can quickly become dehydrated and hypothermic following diarrhea or other illnesses, conditions that alone are life-threatening. The presence and severity of dehydration can be assessed by examination of the stool, urine, and skin. Animals without diarrhea should have well-formed, moist stool pellets. Stools that are dry or smaller than usual may indicate dehydration is occurring. Similarly, urine that is dark in color or scant in amount should be investigated. For a more clinical assessment, a fold of skin on the neck of the animal may be lifted gently, then allowed to return to normal position. If the

TABLE 9. **DRUG DOSAGES FOR GUINEA PIGS**

Drug	Dosage	Route	Indication	Reference
Cefazolin	100 mg/kg BID	IM	Antibiotic	136
Cephalexin	50 mg/kg SID 14D	IM	Antibiotic	137
Chloramphenicol palmitate	50 mg/kg BID 5–7D	PO, SC	Antibiotic	138
Chloramphenicol succinate	30 mg/kg SID 5–7D	IM	Antibiotic	138
Dexamethasone	0.1 mL	SC	Inflammation	137
Diphenhydramine	5 mg/kg	SC	Antihistamine	137
Enrofloxicin	5–10 mg/kg BID 5–7D	PO, SC	Antibiotic	139
Gentamicin	5–8 mg/kg SID	SC	Antibiotic	137
Griseofulvin	15 mg/kg SID 14–28D	PO	Antifungal	124
Heparin	6 mg/kg	IV	Anticoagulant	137
Ivermectin	200–500 (g/kg	SC	Anthelmentic	137,138
Metronidazole	20 mg/kg SID	SC	Antiprotazoal	137
Oxytocin	1–2 units	IM	Stimulate uterus	137
Piperazine Salt	3 mg/ml drinking water	PO	Anthelmintic	138
Sulfamethazine	1 g/liter drinking water 5D	PO	Antibiotic	138
Sulfaquinoxaline	0.1% in drinking water 14D	PO	Coccidiostat	138
Tetracycline	20 mg/kg BID	PO	Antibiotic	137
Trimethoprim — sulfadiazine	30 mg/kg SID	SC	Antibiotic	137

skin fold fails to return to normal position, or takes longer than 1 to 2 seconds to do so, the animal is dehydrated. Hypothermic animals may feel cold to the touch. Taking the temperature with a rectal thermometer will verify an abnormally low core body temperature.

Appropriate replacement fluids should be isotonic, and selected for the animal's condition. Guinea pigs with diarrhea, for example, are probably in need of excess bicarbonate due to an acidotic metabolic state. Fluids are safely and easily administered subcutaneously, but may also be given IP, IV, or intraosseously via the femur.[140] Fluids should be warmed to avoid contributing to hypothermia in debilitated animals. To combat hypothermia, provide sick animals with abundant, dry bedding, heat lamps above the cage, or recirculating warm water blankets. External heat sources such as lamps and blankets must be used carefully and monitored closely to avoid thermal burns and overheating of the animals. Animals that are unable or unwilling to eat may be force-fed, by gavage, a nutrient slurry, or may be given dextrose in fluids as a calorie supplement. In all cases, specific therapy should be directed against a specific etiology.

disease prevention through sanitation

Proper sanitation is imperative to the control of diseases in laboratory animals. Cages and animal rooms should be cleaned and disinfected routinely. Feces, urine, and soiled food and bedding should not be allowed to accumulate in the cage or room. Whenever possible, instruments and equipment should be cleaned and disinfected before being used on another animal. The use of disposable gloves and hand washing with antiseptic soap after handling animals suspected of harboring disease will facilitate control of infectious disease within the facility. Optimally, sick animals should be isolated from healthy animals.

anesthesia and analgesia

The Animal Welfare Act, the PHS Policy, and the Guide all contain requirements for the appropriate use of anesthetics and analgesics for animals in which the proposed procedures may produce more than momentary pain or distress.[83,84,101] This may be accomplished by the judicious use of general (surgical) or local anesthesia, sedation, tranquilization, and/or analgesia.

General anesthesia is a state of temporary, controlled, and reliable unconsciousness with adequate analgesia and muscle relaxation to allow surgical manipulations. Local anesthesia is the loss of sensation to a limited area of the body produced by the injection of a local anesthetic agent. Sedation is a calm state usually associated with drowsiness and mild depression. Tranquilization is a state of relaxation and lack of concern without analgesia or drowsiness. Analgesia is the loss of sensation to pain without the loss of consciousness

Principles of General Anesthesia

General anesthesia should be used for any procedure involving more than momentary pain. Numerous factors may affect the choice of anesthetic used. These include the age of the animal, the health status of the animal, procedure being performed, the length of time the animal needs to be anesthetized, and the potential for drug interaction with the research protocol. All anesthetics used for surgical procedures should be limited to only the amount absolutely necessary to maintain an adequate plane of anesthesia. This may involve gaseous agents, injectable agents, or a combination of these agents. A number of commonly used anesthetic agents for guinea pigs are listed in Table 10. Reversal agents for these anesthetics are listed in Table 11. Abbreviations for route of administration are PO (oral), IV (intravenous), IM (intramuscular), SC (subcutaneous), and IP (intraperitoneal).

Characteristics of Commonly Used Injectable Anesthetics

Continued general anesthesia is difficult to maintain in the guinea pig. A good understanding of anesthetic agents and careful selection of these agents can prevent many problems. To assist in this selection, a brief description of commonly used injectable anesthetic agents along with their associated advantages and disadvantages, indications, and additional useful information are outlined below.

TABLE 10. GENERAL ANESTHETIC AGENTS FOR GUINEA PIGS

Agent	Dosage	Route	Comments	Reference
Atropine sulfate	0.1–2.0 mg/kg	SC	Preanesthetic Anticholinergic	138
Ketamine	40–250 mg/kg	IM	Variable	141
Ketamine + Xylazine	25–80mg/kg+ 0.15–13mg/kg	IM	Variable, lasts 30–60 min	141
Ketamine + Diazepam	44 mg/kg + 0.1 mg/kg	IM		141
Ketamine + Acepromazine	38.3 mg/kg + 1.7 mg/kg	IM		141
Diazepam + Fentanyl	5 mg/kg + 0.32 mg/kg	IP + IM	Increased blood pressure	142
Droperidol + Fentanyl	10–15mg/kg+ 0.2–0.3 mg/kg	IM	Possible tissue damage	141
Methohexital	31 mg/kg	IP		137
Pentobarbital	15–35 mg/kg	IV, IP	Lasts 2 hours	138,141
Tiletamine + Zolazepam	10–80 mg/kg	IM	Lasts 15–30 minutes	141
Ketamine + Xylazine + Methoxyflurane	87 mg/kg + 13 mg/kg + to effect	IM, mask	Variable length of duration	141
Halothane	2–3%	Mask	Gas	141
Methoxyflurane	2%	Chamber mask	Gas	141
Isoflurane	1.15%	Chamber	Gas	141

TABLE 11. REVERSAL AGENTS FOR COMMON ANESTHETICS

Agent	Dosage	Route	Reverses	Reference
Atipamezole	1 mg/kg	IM, IV, IP, SC	Xylazine	143
Doxapram	5–15 mg/kg	IM, IV, IP, SC	Respiratory depression	137
Naloxone	0.01–0.1 mg/kg	IV, IM, IP	Opioids	137
Yohimbine	1.0 mg/kg	IP	Xylazine	144

Atropine

- Preanesthetic agent.

- Anticholinergic activity — decrease salivation and pulmonary secretions, decrease vagal induced bradycardia.

- Promotes cardiac conduction abnormalities.[145,146]

Ketamine

- Dissociative anesthetic.

- Produces catalepsy without good analgesia

- Poor muscle relaxant — skeletal muscle tone increased.

- Frequently used in conjunction with other agents such as xylazine and diazepam.

- Metabolized by the liver and excreted by the kidneys.[145,177]

Xylazine

- Alpha$_2$-adrenergic agonist.

- Potent sedative with analgesic action

- Respiratory and cardiovascular depression

- May produce hyperglycemia and diuresis.[145,147]

Methohexital

- Barbiturate.

- Short duration of action — 2 to 5 minutes.

- Smooth and rapid induction.

- Muscle tremors during recovery.

- Good anesthetic induction agent.

- Respiratory depression.[145]

Pentobarbital

- Barbiturate.

- Produces severe cardiovascular and respiratory depression.

- Effective dose is near the lethal dose.

- Metabolized by the liver.[175]

Fentanyl and droperidol

- Neuroleptanesthesia

- Profound analgesia.

- Moderate respiratory depression

- Mild cardiovascular depression.

- Poor degree of muscle relaxation.

- Hypotension and bradycardia possible.

- Side effects easily prevented with atropine.[148]

Principles of Gas Anesthesia

A review of the guinea pig respiratory system should be undertaken before gas anesthetics are used.[149] Administration of gas anesthetic, alone or in combination with injectable agent(s), provides an excellent way to control the length and depth of anesthesia. It is also easier to provide supplemental oxygen and ventilate the animal while using anesthetic gas. Use of an endotracheal tube, face mask, or nose cone are methods of providing gas anesthesia to guinea pigs. Excellent reviews of the principles of gas anesthesia may be found elsewhere.[145,146]

Gas anesthesia requires the use of specialized equipment. The anesthetic machine used for guinea pigs may be the same as that used for cats and dogs or it may be specially made for rodents (Figure 34). To further administer the gaseous anesthetic, a face mask complete with a diaphragm that seals around the face (Figure 35) or an endotracheal tube are needed. Some

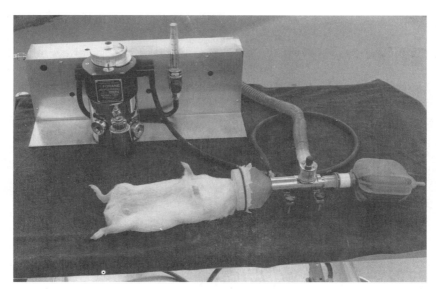

FIG. 34.   Model 4001MSG Vetamac table top anesthetic machine complete with two flowmeters and pop-off valve for efficient waste gas scavenging.

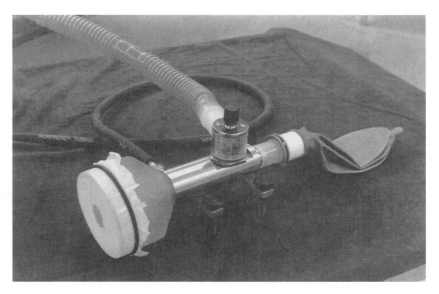

FIG. 35.   Model 4003 Vetamac small rodent manifold for anesthetic gas delivery with non-rebreathing circuit and airtight diaphragm.

gaseous anesthetic agents, such as methoxyflurane, may also be administered to guinea pigs via a nose cone, which can be made from an empty 12 mL syringe case with anesthetic soaked cotton in the end, or in a bell jar with a tight sealing lid. Disadvantages of these last two methods of administrations are lack of control of the depth of anesthesia and use of an appropriate hood to remove waste gas. A scavenger system for waste gas for the anesthetic machine is also a necessity. This may be a permanent method or disposable gas traps may be purchased and added to the equipment.

Endotracheal intubation of the guinea pig can prove difficult. Recommended tube size is 1.5 to 2.5 mm outside diameter (OD) for a 400 to 1000 g guinea pig.[137] Methods for making endotracheal tubes for guinea pigs from a catheter or plastic tubing have also been described.[150,151] If the use of a face mask seems better suited to the situation, it made be made following directions published elsewhere, or purchased from a commercial vendor.[152,153]

characteristics of commonly used gas anesthetics

Halothane

- Halogenated hydrocarbon anesthetic.

- Good muscular relaxation.

- Rapid induction and recovery.

- Respiratory and cardiovascular depression.

- Sensitizes heart to arrhythmias.

- Metabolized by the liver with microsomal enzyme induction.[145,148]

Methoxyflurane

- Halogenated hydrocarbon anesthetic.

- Potent anesthetic with post-operative analgesia

- Slow induction and recovery time.

- Mild to moderate respiratory and cardiovascular depression.
- Fluoride ion release that may induce renal and hepatic damage.[145,148]

Isoflurane

- Rapid induction and recovery.
- Depth of anesthesia easily altered.
- Severe respiratory depression, mild to moderate cardiovascular depression.
- Little biotransformation, therefore, little effect on liver and kidneys.
- Good anesthetic for drug metabolism and toxicology studies.[145]

Principles of Local Anesthesia

A portion or specific area of the body may be rendered insensitive to pain with the use of local anesthetics. These agents are frequently used for minor procedures or for those involving the skin and subcutaneous tissue. These agents may be injected into the tissues or the epidural space or directly applied to the skin or eye. A description of epidural catheter placement in the guinea pig has been published.[154] Characteristics of commonly used local anesthetics follow:

Lidocaine

- Good local and epidural anesthetic
- Infusion of a small volume, 0.5 to 2 mL of a 2% solution, by needle, 25 gauge, and syringe into or around the area of interest.
- Normal doses have no adverse effects, however, high doses may produce adverse cardiovascular effects.
- Additive effect with other antiarrhythmic drugs.[155]

Proparacaine

- 0.5% ophthalmic solution.

- Good local anesthesia of the eye and surrounding tissues.

- Applied as a drop to the eye and allowed to remain for one to five minutes, then removed from eye by tilting the guinea pig.

Sedation and Tranquilization of Guinea Pigs

Guinea pigs that are hard to handle may need to be sedated or tranquilized. These agents may also be used as preanesthetic agents or in conjunction with anesthetics to produced balanced anesthesia. Commonly used sedatives and tranquilizers used in guinea pigs are listed in Table 12.

TABLE 12. COMMON SEDATIVES/TRANQUILIZERS FOR GUINEA PIGS

Agent	Dosage	Route	Indication	Reference
Acepromazine	1–2 mg/kg	IM	Preanesthetic, tranquilizer	137
Chlorpromazine	0.2 mg/kg	SC	Preanesthetic, tranquilizer	137
Diazepam	2.5–5 mg/kg	IP, IM	Sedative	137
Xylazine	3–5 mg/kg	IM	Preanesthetic, sedative	137

Analgesia

In keeping with the appropriate use of anesthetics, sedatives, and tranquilizers, the use of analgesics to control pain and discomfort during and after procedures, is imperative. It may be assumed, unless there is evidence to the contrary, that any procedure that would produce pain in humans will produce pain in guinea pigs. Another point to remember is that it is best to prevent pain where it is likely to occur.

Guinea pigs are very stoic animals and frequently there are very few, if any, indicators of pain. Signs of pain in the guinea pig might include decreased food and water consumption, change in behavior, change in activity level, and utterance of sharp, harsh, high-pitched squeals when handled or manipulated.[16,156] Table 13 contains a list of common analgesics for use in the guinea pig.

TABLE 13. COMMONLY USED ANALGESICS FOR GUINEA PIGS

Agent	Dosage	Route	Duration	Reference
Aspirin	86 mg/kg	PO	4 hrs	137
Buprenorphine	0.05–0.06 mg/kg	IM, SC	8–12 hrs	137, 157
Butorphanol	0.025–0.4 mg/kg	IM, SC	4–12 hrs	157
Ibuprofen	10 mg/kg	IM	4 hrs	137
Meperidine	10–20 mg/kg	IM, SC	2–3 hrs	137
Morphine	2–10 mg/kg	IM, SC	2–4 hrs	137
Phenylbutazone	40 mg/kg	PO		137

Perianesthetic Management

General anesthesia can lead to numerous physiologic changes and potential complications. To correct these changes and reduce the incidence of complications, the following recommendations are made.

preanesthetic care

- Only healthy, purpose-bred guinea pigs from a known, reputable vendor should be used.

- Each animal should receive a physical examination including general appearance; behavior; body temperature (if possible); and color of mucous membranes of mouth, eye, and perineum. Animals with an elevated temperature or pale or bright-red mucous membranes are not good candidates for surgery. Auscultation of the chest and abdomen, listening for abnormal heart or lung sounds should be performed. Care should be taken to examine the animal for signs of disease, such as diarrhea and nasal discharge. Any guinea pig with abnormal heart or lung sounds or clinical signs of disease should not be used for surgical procedures.

- If possible, basic hematological parameters should be monitored. This may not always be possible due to procedural design and animal size. Animals with results outside the normal range, such as an elevated white blood cell count, low hematocrit, or elevated BUN, should probably not be used for a surgical procedure.

- The exact weight of the animal should be obtained for accurate dosing of anesthetic agents.

- Guinea pigs do not need to be fasted before anesthesia or surgery, except if performing procedures on the gastrointestinal tract.

- Preanesthetic treatment with atropine, 0.1 to 2.0 mg/kg IM, is useful in reducing respiratory and gastrointestinal secretions. Glycopyrrolate may be used in place of atropine as an anticholinergic.

- Warmed subcutaneous fluids, lactated Ringer's solution, 0.9% saline, or 5% glucose, should be administered during surgical procedures at the rate of 10 to 15 mL/kg of body weight per hour of procedural duration.

- Due to the loss of palpebral reflexes, the cornea may dry out during an extended procedure. Ophthalmic ointment should be placed into each eye during anesthesia.

anesthetic care

- During the course of anesthesia, the depth of anesthesia and physiological character of the anesthetized animal should be monitored frequently.

- There are four stages of anesthesia. These are used in the evaluation of anesthetic depth.[176]

  Stage I — Loss of pain without the loss of consciousness.

  Stage II — Loss of consciousness that may include struggling and whining with many reflexes still present.

  Stage III — Surgical anesthesia with loss of reflexes, muscle relaxation, and rhythmic, deep breathing. Planes 1 to 4, mild to deep, are used to further evaluate this stage.

  Stage IV — Medullary paralysis with respiratory arrest, hypotension, and imminent death.

> **Note:** Stage IV is to be avoided. The animal is too deeply anesthetized.

- Numerous reflexes should be used to evaluate the depth of anesthesia before a procedure is begun and throughout the procedure.

  The pedal reflex is monitored by firmly pinching a toe while the leg is extended. If a surgical stage of anesthesia has been reached, the guinea pig will make no attempt to withdraw the limb, however, this response is variable between animals.

  The ear pinch reflex is monitored by firmly pinching the ear of the guinea pig. The animal will flinch if a surgical plane of anesthesia has not been reached.

  The jaw tone of the guinea pigs is also an indication of the depth of anesthesia. The jaw will resist opening if the animal is too lightly anesthetized.

- Changes in the rhythm and rate of respiration and heart rate may indicate a change in depth of anesthesia. Some animals have increased respiratory and heart rates when pain insensation is insufficient.

- Cardiovascular function should be evaluated via examination of mucous membranes of the eye, nose, mouth, and perineum. These should remain pink in color and moist. A darkening or bluish color indicates a lack of proper oxygenation of these areas and, therefore, poor circulatory function. This may also be evaluated via electrocardiogram (ECG) and blood gas levels and pH.

- A small animal like a guinea pig can lose body heat very easily during anesthesia. To prevent this, animals should be maintained on a warm surface, such as towels and a recirculating water pad, and not placed directly onto the surface of a stainless steel table. Care should be taken to avoid thermal burns to the animal.[158]

- Judicious administration of warmed fluids can also be used to maintain body heat and improve cardiovascular function.

Note: Although reflexes are a good indication of the depth of anesthesia, it is possible for the occasional guinea pig to not lose all reflexes under surgical anesthesia. Close attention should be paid to all evaluations of anesthetic depth, including, respiration, mucous membrane color, and anesthetic dose given compared to animal weight.

---

postanesthetic care

- Postanesthetic care is a critical time in the recovery of the animal. Monitoring of the parameters described above should continue until the guinea pig is fully recovered.

- Place the guinea pig in a clean, dry cage, with a small amount of bedding, without food and water until the animal has recovered from anesthesia and is easily moving about.

- Monitor the body temperature and provide appropriate supplemental heat.

- Monitor the color of mucous membranes.

- Monitor heart and respiratory rate and character.

- Administer warmed subcutaneous fluids if needed.

Note: If recovery time is protracted, consult a qualified veterinarian.

---

aseptic surgery

The AWA, PHS Policy, and Guide require that surgery on guinea pigs be performed using aseptic conditions and techniques.[83,84,101] This does not require a separate surgery room, however, a dedicated surgery area that remains clutter-free, is easily sanitized, and is used only for surgery, is required. Extensive descriptions of aseptic techniques have been described elsewhere.[159-162] Briefly, these procedures involve the following:

- Shave a generous area around the surgical site with electric clippers.

- Clean and scrub the skin at the surgical site with an antiseptic. Start along the proposed incision line and move outward in a circular motion.

- Isolate the surgical area with sterile drapes.

- Sterile instruments should be used for all procedures.

- Surgeons and assistants should were sterile gloves, surgery gowns, face masks, and caps.

- All personnel performing and assisting with the procedures should be properly trained in sterile and surgical techniques.

postsurgical management

Following a surgical procedure, the guinea pigs should be closely monitored until fully recovered from anesthesia. Then the animal should be checked frequently, monitoring for signs of possible complications.

- The behavior of the guinea pigs should be followed, as it was before the procedure began, to look for signs of pain or other abnormalities.

- The edges of the surgical incision should be checked for apposition and signs of animal chewing on the area. If the guinea pig begins to bother the area, a cervical collar (Figure 36) may be placed on the animal. Tissue glue may be used to reappose the surgical edges if the open area is not too large.

- The guinea pigs should be closely monitored for signs of infection including:

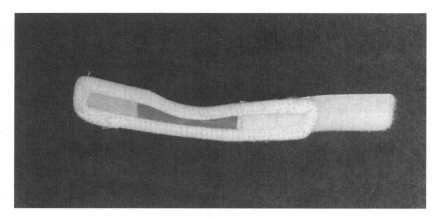

FIG. 36.   Guinea pig cervical collar for prevention and treatment of self-inflicted trauma.

1.   Oozing from the surgical incision of yellow, white, or green material.

2.   Abnormal swelling, heat, or redness of the area.

3.   Elevated body temperature.

4.   Any discharge should be cultured and appropriate antibiotic therapy, under the guidance of a qualified veterinarian, begun.

euthanasia

Euthanasia is the act of inducing humane death in animals without the occurrence of pain or distress. Guinea pigs should be euthanized at the end of the study, when there is severe illness or disability, or when there is intractable pain. The method chosen should induce loss of consciousness and death without causing pain, anxiety, or distress. The method should be reliable, safe for personnel, irreversible, and compatible with the purpose or requirements of the study. It is well documented that the method of euthanasia can physiologically alter the animal.[163-165] Death of the guinea pig should be confirmed by opening the thoracic cavity, cutting the diaphragm, removing the heart, or closely monitoring the heart beat with a stethoscope. Effective methods of euthanasia of guinea pigs are found

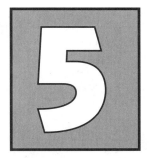

experimental methodology

Many research projects involve the use of guinea pigs, however, it is beyond the scope of this book to detail all of these, therefore, only a few of the more commonly used procedures will be decribed here. Before any new procedure or research project is started, all personnel involved must be properly trained in those procedures, as well as proper equipment acquired.

restraint

Guinea pigs are docile and easily handled animals. They frequently squeal when being handled and ocassionally struggle and bite. Most guinea pigs will "stampede" when being caught or stand still until the last second and then flee just before being grasped. To reduce this flight response and possible injuries to the animal and frustration to personnel, it is best to approach a guinea pig as quietly and slowly as possible.[167]

Manual restraint
This is the most common method used with guinea pigs. When handling and restraining a guinea pig the following should be remembered:

- The guinea pig should be grasped firmly and carefully aroung the chest with both hands. Young guinea pigs may be grasped with just one hand.

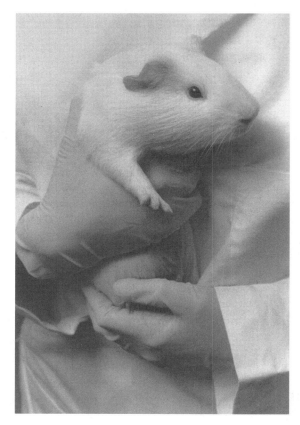

FIG. 37.   Proper manual restraint of a large guinea pig with one hand on the chest and the other hand supporting the hindquarters.

- The guinea pig has a very small chest for the size of the animal and care must be taken to not squeeze the chest too firmly for too long. Too tight a grasp may make it impossible for the animal to breathe.

- Large, pregnant sows or heavy boars also will need to have the rear quarters supported with one hand while being held to prevent injury (Figure 37).

- Simple procedures may be performed by holding the guinea pig firmly against the body or with the head held in the crook of the elbow.

- The guinea pig may be restrained by holding the chest and forelegs in one hand and the pelvis and hindlegs in the other hand.

- The guinea pig may also be restrained for simple procedures by holding the anterior portion of the animal up by the chest while allowing the rear legs to remain on the surface supporting the animal.

- Most guinea pigs become accustomed to being handled and will eventually flee and struggle less.

Restraint Devices

Restraint devices are available for guinea pigs, however, they are infrequently used nor necessary.[168]

sampling techniques

The compact size and shape of the guinea pig make it more difficult than other animals to sample blood and other bodily fluids, however, many sites are accessible for sampling, provided you have the proper knowledge.

Blood Collection

Blood is frequently required for numerous research projects involving guinea pigs, such as production of polycloncal antibodies and collection of complement for *in vito* assays. It is also necessary to collect blood and submit it for testing for viral diseases in guinea pig colonies or when animals are housed for prolonged periods of time.

- The **volume** of blood that may be collected depends upon the size of the guinea pig and the time interval between collections. If blood is removed too quickly the animal may suffer hypovolemic shock, while if too much blood is removed, the animal may become severely anemic. As a general rule, 10% of the circulating blood volume may be removed every three to four weeks. The recommendation for daily, or less, sampling is 1% of the blood volume, which will produce minimal adverse effects to the animal.[169] The average blood volume of a guinea pig is 75 mL/kg, therefore, 6.5 to 7.7 mL/kg of body weight could be removed every 3 to 4 weeks.[137,170]

- Appropriate **sampling** vials should be used. Vials containing an anticoagulant, such as EDTA, are used for whole blood for cellular analysis, such as CBC, complete blood cell count for red cell parameters, and white blood cell differential count. However, for the collection of plasma, whole blood is collected into vials containing either heparin, citrate, or potassium oxalate. Blood samples collected for serum chemistry are collected into vials that contain nothing, or contain a clot accelerator. Serum samples may be obtained quickly by using an empty vial for blood collection and centrifuging the vial at 800 to 1000 × g for 10 to 15 minutes. The liquid portion in the vial is the serum. However, the same result is obtained when the vial is left still at room temperature for 30 to 60 minutes.

The more commonly used blood sampling techniques and sites are described below:

Percutaneous blood sampling should follow these general guidelines:

- Collection usually involves the use of a disposable needle and syringe to puncture the skin and access a blood vessel.

- The diameter (gauge) of the needle should be slightly smaller than the diameter of the vessel to be accessed.

- Needles and syringes should be disposed of after only one use. The entire syringe with attached needle should be placed in a designated plastic container for sharp objects. To prevent puncture wounds to personnel, the needle cap should not be replaced over the needle before disposal.[104]

The **site** for percutaneous blood sampling should be chosen based upon the size of the guinea pig and the volume of blood needed. Large volumes of blood may be collected from the anterior or posterior vena cava or the heart;

moderate volumes of blood from the peripheral vessels of the legs and ears, the dorsolateral penile vein, and the retro-orbital sinus; and small amounts of blood may be obtained by clipping a toenail very short. When repeated sampling is necessary, the site of collection should be rotated.

The **anterior vena cava** may be used as a survival method for the collection of a large quantity (refer to previous section on appropriate blood volume). Hemorrhage and cardiac tamponade are major risks for this procedure.[171,172]

➤ *Procedure*

1. Anesthetize the guinea pig and place it in dorsal recumbancy.

2. Locate the area of the thoracic inlet on the right side (the guinea pig will be upside down). This is the area at the junction of the uppermost portion of the sternum and the first rib (Figure 38).

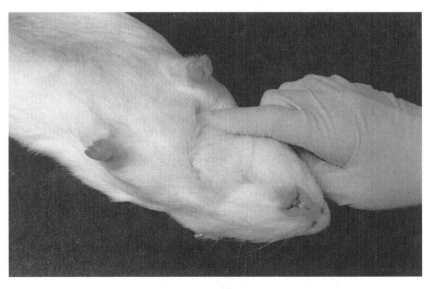

FIG. 38. Location of the thoracic inlet, dorsal to the junction of the uppermost portion of the sternum and the first rib, for anterior vena cava blood collection.

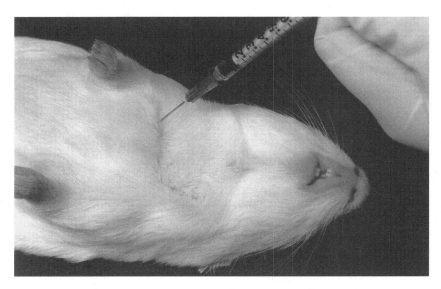

Fig. 39. Appropriate insertion of the needle for blood collection from or injection into the anterior vena cava.

3. Insert the needle, 22 to 25 gauge $^5/_8$-1", at a 30 to 45°angle while slowly pulling back on the plunger (Figure 39).

4. The needle is directed towards the midline of the thorax to a depth of 10 to 16 mm.

5. When blood appears in the hub of the needle, draw back on the plunger and collect the required volume.

6. Apply pressure to the site upon needle removal to prevent the formation of a hematoma.

Cardiocentesis (intracardiac blood collection) may also be used for the collection of a large amount of blood. It carries the same risks upon recovery as does the anterior vena cava procedure.

➤ *Procedure*

1. Anesthetize the guinea pig and place it in right lateral recumbancy, right side down.

2. Palpate the area of the strongest heartbeat over the ribs on the animal's left side. This area may also be

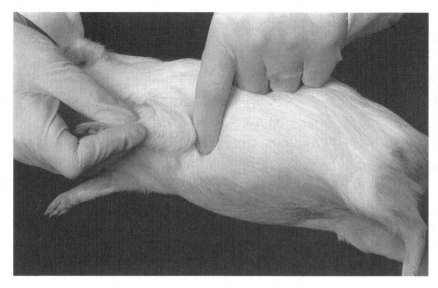

Fig. 40   Location of the strongest heartbeat area at the point of the elbow in the flexed left forelimb. This is the appropriate location for cardiocentesis.

    located by flexing the front leg and feeling at the
    area located at the point of the elbow (Figure 40).

3. Insert the needle, 20 to 25 gauge 1 to $1^1/_2$",
    perpendicular to and between the guinea pig's ribs
    (Figure 41).

4. Slowly withdraw the plunger until blood appears in
    the hub, then withdraw the desired volume.

5. An alternative method for the collection of blood
    from the heart is to place the guinea pig in dorsal
    recumbancy, insert the needle at a 30 to 45°angle
    under the sternum just left of the midline
    (Figure 42).[171]

6. Cardiocentesis is considered a nonsurvival procedure
    by some experts, however, it has been used
    successfully as a survival procedure by others.[171]

The posterior vena cava may be used to collect moderate to large amounts of blood, however, the results are not as consistent as the two previous methods.

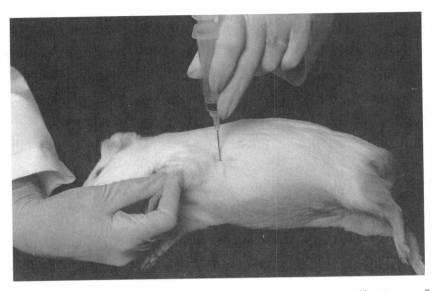

Fig. 41. Appropriate needle placement for the collection of blood from or injection of compounds into the heart.

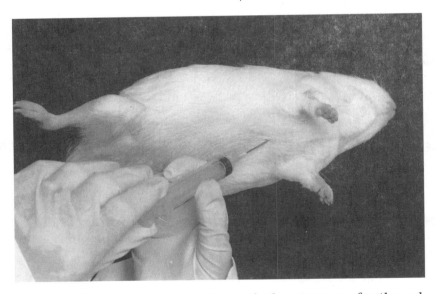

Fig. 42. Alternative method, beneath the sternum, for the collection of blood from the heart of a guinea pig.

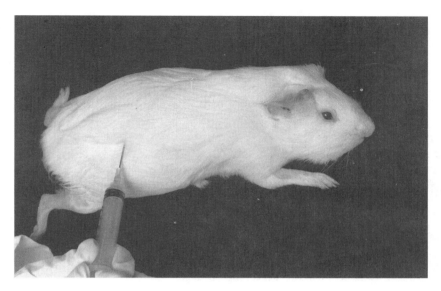

FIG. 43.   Appropriate method for the collection of blood from the posterior vena cava. The needle should be inserted perpendicular to the guinea pig just below the spinal column and behind the last rib.

➤ Procedure

1. Anesthetize the guinea pig and place it in ventral recumbancy.

2. Insert the needle on the right side of the guinea pig, parallel to the resting surface and perpendicular to the animal, below the vertebral column and caudal to the junction of the last rib (Figure 43).

3. Slowly withdraw the plunger while inserting the needle until blood is observed in the needle hub. Then withdraw the desired volume.

The **retro-orbital sinus** of the guinea pig may be used to collecte moderate to large volumes of blood.[171]

➤ Procedure

1. Anesthetize the guinea pig and place in ventral recumbancy.

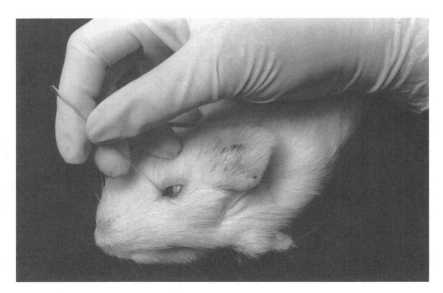

Fig. 44. Appropriate placement of the hematocrit tube for the collection of blood from the retro-orbital sinus.

2. Place a hematocrit tube at the medial canthus of the eye beside the globe (Figure 44).

3. While rotating the tube, apply enough pressure to insert the tube through the membrane.

4. Continue to rotate the tube and apply pressure until the tube begins to fill with blood.

5. Many hematocrit tubes may be filled at this time or flow may allow dripping into tubes.

6. Apply pressure to the area when finished to insure proper hemostasis.

The **femoral vessels** may be used to collect moderate to large volumes of blood.[173]

➤ *Procedure*

1. The guinea pig may be tranquilized, held in a restrainer, manually restrained, or anesthetized and placed in dorsal recumbancy.

2. Locate the femoral triangle (the area just caudal to the midline of the hairless rim of the last inguinal nipple).

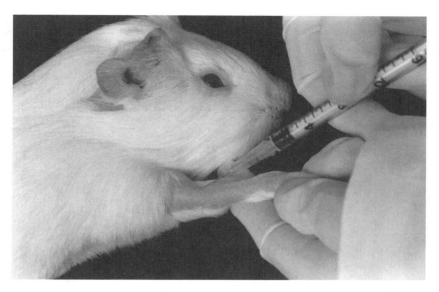

Fig. 45. Collection of blood from the cephalic vein. This site may also be used for injections.

3. Insert the needle, 23 gauge $^3/_4$", at a 45°angle to a depth of about $^1/_4$".

4. Slowly retract the plunger until blood begins to flow, then collect the desired volume.

5. Apply digital pressure to the area after needle withdrawal to ensure adequate hemostasis.

6. This sample is collected blindly resulting in approximately 60% aterial blood samples and 40% venous samples.

Numerous other percutaneous sites may be used for the collection of small to moderate volumes of blood:

- Medial saphenous vein.[174]

- Lateral metatarsal vein.[175]

- Auricular veins. These veins may be used for repeated collections using a lancet.[176,177]

- Cephalic vein (Figure 45).[178]

- Dorsolateral penile vein.[167]

- Footpad.[179]

The carotid artery and jugular vein may be used for the collection of blood, however, these procedures usually require surgical exposure of the vessels.[173]

The **method for percutaneous** blood collection

➤ *Technique*

- In many instances it is easier to observe blood vessels and obtain a blood sample if the fur has been removed from the area with electric clippers.

- Scrub the skin with an antiseptic such as 70% isopropyl alcohol.

- Visually locate the vessel of interest, if possible.

- Withdraw the plunger slightly before inserting into the guinea pig to break the airlock in the syringe.

- Insert the needle with the beveled edge up.

- Slowly withdraw the plunger during insertion of the needle. When blood is observed within the hub of the needle, then the desired site has probably been reached.

- Withdraw blood with light and steady pressure. If too much pressure is used and the plunger withdrawn too quickly, the vessel may collapse and halt blood flow.

- If blood flow is interrupted, and the plunger is not being withdrawn too quickly, rotate the needle slightly. Slight changes in the needle orientation will usually restart the flow of blood.

- At the end of the procedure, maintain digital pressure to the area to prevent hematoma formation and maintain adequate hemostasis.

Indwelling catheters have been used in guinea pigs for the collection of multiple blood samples and repeated intravenous injections. This usually requires surgical exposure of the vessel in the guinea pig.

- **Sites** for placement of catheters include:
  - Carotid artery.[180]
  - Jugular vein.[173]

- Vascular access ports may be used with guinea pigs for chronic access to vessels, however, because of the anatomy and research protocols, they are infrequently used.

Urine Collection

The collection of urine from guinea pigs may be accomplished by use of one of a number of methods. The method chosen will depend upon the volume needed, need for lack of contamination, and period of time for which urine needs to be collected. Urine samples should be kept under refrigeration until analyzed to prevent bacterial overgrowth.

- **Manual manipulation** of the urinary bladder by applying pressure over the caudal abdominal area near the midline. A stream of urine should be produced, however, care should be taken to not apply too much pressure and rupture the urinary bladder.[181] This will provide a relatively clean urine sample, however, it may become contaminated via the animals fur.

- A **metabolism cage** may be purchased from a commercial vendor and used for the collection and separation of urine and feces over longer periods of time. Urine may become contaminated during this process.

- A **surgical method** for the chronic catheterization of the urinary bladder for rodents has been described. This method allows for the continuous collection of uncontaminated urine from the conscious animal.[182]

- **Cystocentesis** may be used to collect uncontaminated urine. A needle, with attached syringe, is inserted into the urinary bladder through the abdominal wall. The guinea pig should be prepared as if this was a surgical procedure. The needle is inserted into the bladder at the midline of the animal in the caudal abdomen just cranial to the pubis. The plunger is withdrawn and urine should begin to appear in the syringe.

- Urine may be collected from the cage floor or in the pan beneath a suspended cage, if contamination is not a problem.

Milk Collection

The collection of milk from nursing sows has been described.[181,183] The technique involves construction and use of a miniature milking machine. Up to 9.0 mL can be collected from a large sow.[211,213] A method has also been developed for the collection of small samples of milk from multiple biopsies of the mammary glands of guinea pigs during pregnancy and lactation.[184]

compound administration techniques

The administration of compounds can be accomplished via many different routes. The guinea pig should be firmly restrained, tranquilized, sedated, or anesthetized before administration to reduce pain and distress and facilitate proper administration techniques.

Intravascular (IV)

Intravascular administration is widely used, but in the guinea pig the access to veins is somewhat difficult. However, this does not preclude the use of this method and, in fact, this may frequently be the method of choice for delivery of numerous liquid substances.

Many of the common sites for intravascular administration are the same as those for the collection of blood and include:

- The **auricular veins** of the ears may be used for intravascular administration.
- Anterior vena cava.[177]
- Medial saphenous vein.[174]
- Lateral metatarsal vein.[175]

The technique for the administration of liquids via intravascular administration is as follows:

➤ *Technique*

1. Shave and prepare the area as for blood collection.

2. While inserting the needle, withdraw the plunger slowly. When blood is observed in the hub, withdraw the plunger further. The appearance of blood within the syringe will ensure proper placement within the vein.

3. Slowly inject the solution. The formation of a raised area surrounding or near the needle is an indication that the needle has come out of the vein, and the injection needs to be stopped.

4. A blanching, light coloration that replaces the red coloration of the vein, will be observed during proper administration in superficial veins.

5. Watch the guinea pig closely for signs of an adverse reaction to the compound, such as increase in respiration rate. Stop injection if this occurs.

6. Apply digital pressure to the area to ensure proper hemostasis and to prevent hematoma formation.

➤ *Procedure*

1. Firmly restrain the guinea pig. Restraint devices for this procedure have been described.[168,177]

2. Sedation of the guinea pig with acepromazine (1 to 2 mg/kg IM) may be used to dilate the vessels. The vessels may also be dilated by warming the guinea pig under a lamp (Figure 46). Be careful not to burn the animal.

3. While holding the ear taut, insert the needle (25 to 26 gauge ⅝") almost parallel to the ear (Figure 47).[176]

4. Withdraw the plunger slowly while inserting the needle, being careful not to apply too much pressure or the vein will collapse. Once blood is seen in the hub, then slowly inject compound.

Indwelling intravascular catheters, as with blood collection, may be placed in the jugular vein, carotid artery, aorta, and ventricles for chronic intravascular administration of compounds.[180,185]

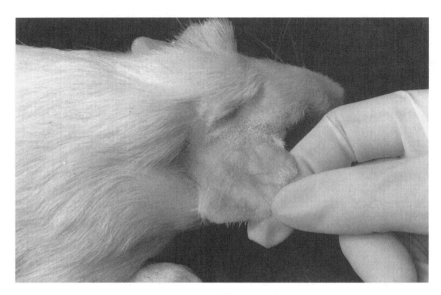

FIG. 46.   Dilated auricular vessels of the ear of a guinea pig.

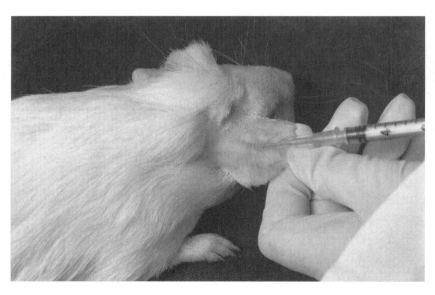

FIG. 47.   Appropriate method for the injection of substances or collection of blood from the guinea pig ear. The marginal vessels may also be used.

Intramuscular (IM)

Intramuscular administration of compounds is an easy method, however, the volume that may be given is limited. The gluteal muscles of the hindlimb are the most frequently used in the guinea pig.[171]

➤ Procedure

1. Review the anatomy of the guinea pig hindlimb so that major vessels and the sciatic nerve may be avoided.

2. Firmly restrain the guinea pig and immobilize the rear limb.

3. Clean the area with alcohol or an antiseptic.

4. Insert the needle (22 to 30 gauge) into the muscle mass at a 30°angle (Figure 48).

5. Withdraw the plunger slowly. If blood appears in the needle hub, withdraw the needle and insert it again through the skin and into the muscle mass.

6. Inject the compound in a steady motion, not too fast. For a large volume, several sites may need to be used. No more than 0.3 mL should be injected into each IM site.[137]

Subcutaneous (SC)

Subcataneous administration of compounds is an easy method for delivery of large volumes (5 to 10 mL).[137] The subcutis of the dosum (top) of the back is the most frequently used site.[171]

➤ Procedure

1. Firmly restrain the guinea pig and place on a firm surface.

2. Grasp the nape of the neck with the thumb and forefinger.

3. Clean the area with an antiseptic.

4. Insert the needle (22 to 30 gauge) at the base of the skin fold between the thumb and forefinger (Figure 49).

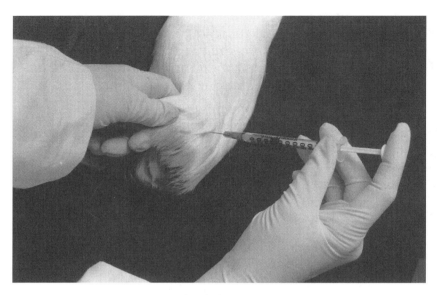

FIG. 48. Appropriate method for intramuscular injection into the gluteal muscles of a guinea pig. Care should be taken to avoid the sciatic nerve.

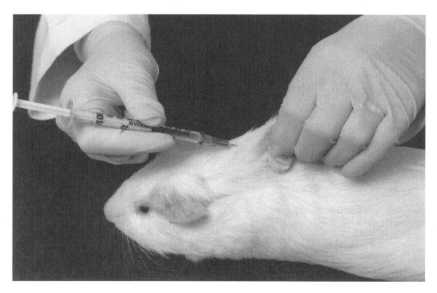

FIG. 49. Appropriate method for subcutaneous injection in the guinea pig. A skinfold is held between the thumb and forefinger while the needle is inserted and substance injected.

5. Slowly withdraw the plunger. If blood is seen in the needle hub, withdraw the needle and replace in skinfold.

6. Inject compound with a steady motion. More than one site should be used if the injection volume is very large.

Intraperitoneal (IP)

Intraperitoneal injecion of compounds is also useful for large volumes (10 to 15 mL).[137] However, the risk of puncture of the intestines or urinary bladder and possible peritonitis are present.[171]

➤ *Procedure*

1. Firmly restrain the guinea pig by holding the animal's thorax in one hand and the pelvis in the other. Hold the animal upright in a vertical position.

2. Insert the needle at a 30°angle into the lower right quadrant of the abdomen (Figure 50).

3. Slowly withdraw the plunger. The appearance of blood or other fluid in the needle hub indicates improper placement. Withdraw the needle and try again.

4. Inject compound with a steady motion.

Intradermal (ID)

Intradermal injection is sometimes used as a delivery method for compounds for toxicity testing or other immunologic protocols.[171]

➤ *Procedure*

1. Firmly restrain or anesthetize the guinea pig and place the animal in ventral recumbancy.

2. Shave the fur on the back and scrub the area with an antiseptic.

3. With the bevel up, insert the needle between the layers of skin at a 20°angle (Figure 51).

4. Slowly withdraw the plunger. The appearance of blood or other fluids in the needle hub indicates inproper placement. Withdraw the needle and replace.

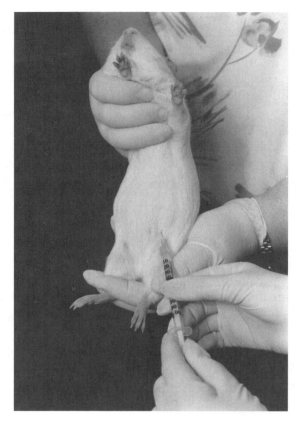

Fig. 50. Appropriate method for intraperitoneal injection in the guinea pig. The needle is inserted into the ventral abdomen, lateral to the midline.

5. Inject a small volume, 0.05 mL or less, slowly to form a "bleb", affirm rounded circular skin welt. Repeat at additional sites until the entire dose of compound has been administered.

Implantable **osmotic pumps** may be used for continuous administration of compounds into the subcutis or abdominal cavity. These are small capsule shaped objects designed to deliver compounds at a set rate. Different rate pumps may be obtained. The pump is surgically impanted via a very small incision or a large bore needle.

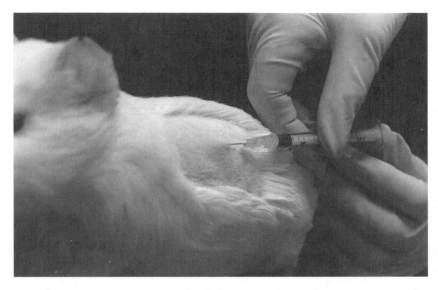

Fig. 51. Appropriate method for intradermal injection in the guinea pig. The needle is inserted between the layers of skin and a small "bleb" is apparent after compound is injected.

Oral (PO)

Several methods for oral (PO) administration of compounds exist for guinea pigs. These methods can be used for the administration of known quantities of liquids, slurries, and semi-solids.

1. Many compounds may be added to the drinking water. However, guinea pigs tend to dislike anything that is new and may not drink at all. Monitor carefully to ensure that the animals are drinking. This method does not provide precise dosing.

2. Numerous compounds may be administered orally by squirting the substance into the back of the mouth. A syringe or dosing needle with a rounded end, which can be purchased commercially, is inserted into the mouth behind the incisor teeth. The compound is then squirted into the mouth, taking care to allow the animal time to swallow. This also is not an exact method.

3. Oral gavage is an exact method for compound administration. A 16 to 18 gauge, 3 to 4" dosing needle with a rounded, ball end is used.[171]

➤ *Procedure*

1. The needle should be measured to assure it is not too long. The needle should reach from mouth to last rib (Figure 52).

2. Firmly restrain guinea pig . Animal may have hind limbs resting on surface or be securely held.

3. Tilt the guinea pig's head towards the ceiling.

4. Insert the needle into the guinea pig's mouth (Figure 53).

5. Slide needle tip down the back of the mouth and into the esophagus. Any resistance felt indicates improper placement of the needle. Needle should slide into the esophagus easily.

6. Improper placement of the needle will result in the placement of the compound within the lungs.

7. Slowly administer the compound. If any changes in respiration occur, such as increased rate or depth, stop immediately, withdraw the needle, and try to reinsert into the esophagus. Too much pressure on the plunger of the syringe may separate the syringe from the needle and waste the compound.

Oral gavage via a gastric tube has also been used in guinea pigs. This method is easier for the administration of a large volume.[181]

➤ *Procedure*

1. Anesthetize the guinea pig.

2. Use a soft rubber or flexible plastic tube 1.5 to 6 mm in diameter.

3. Insert tube into stomach by moistening the end of the tube with water and inserting the tube into the esophagus through the mouth. A mouth gag must be

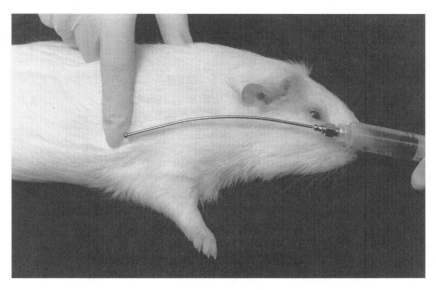

FIG. 52. Measurement of a stainless steel dosing needle. The needle should reach from the mouth to the last rib.

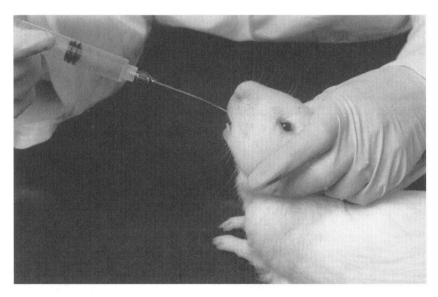

FIG. 53. Appropriate method for the insertion of a dosing needle into the stomach of a guinea pig.

placed into the mouth before passing the tube so that the guinea pig does not bite into the tubing. The gag can be made from a piece of sterilized wood with a hole cut in the center or from a plastic syringe case with the end cut off so that it resembles an open tube. A rush of air coming out of the tube indicates it has been placed in the respiratory system and needs to be removed and replaced within the stomach.

4. Slowly administer the compound. If respiratory distress occurs, stop immediately, kink the tube to prevent leakage of compound, and remove the tube. Reinsert the tube into the stomach and try again.

Intracerebroventricular

Intracerebroventricular administration allows delivery of compounds directly into the brain. Stereotaxic surgery is required for exact placement of the catheters.[186]

Aural — Inner Ear

Chronic delivery of compounds into the inner ear of guinea pigs is possible. A catheter is surgically implanted near the round window membrane of the middle ear. Compounds are instilled there and allowed to diffuse through the membrane. This method can be used for toxicity and efficacy testing of compounds for middle ear infections.[187]

adjuvants

Adjuvants are used in many safety tests to bolster the immune response. Adjuvants are know to produce mild to severe tissue damage.[188] Freund's complete adjuvant (FCA), Freund's incomplete adjuvant (FIA), aluminum phosphate, and trehalose dimycolate are some of the adjuvants used in guinea pigs. A thorough review of the literature and regulations should be undertaken to obtain information of the best and most acceptable adjuvants available and those applicable for current use. Studies have been completed comparing many of these adjuvant products.[189,190]

safety testing procedures

In the analysis of the safety of and potential for hypersensitization to compounds, such as drugs and pesticides, laws and regulations exist regulating the testing of these substances. Certain procedures, stipulated by law, require that guinea pigs be used as the test model.[191,192] These tests include Freund's complete adjuvant test, guinea pig maximization test, split adjuvant test, Buehler test, open epicutaneous test, Mauer optimization test, footpad technique, and general safety test. These tests are precisely described or referenced in the Code for the Federal Register.[193,194]

The following are brief descriptions of the Magnusson maximization test,[195] the Buehler closed-patch sensitization test,[196] and the guinea pig antigenicity (anaphylaxis) test.[197] These tests are performed before approval of products for human use, however, the properties of the test compound and the regulations of the various countries will determine the selection of methods. The Magnusson maximization test is currently required by European regulatory agencies which do not accept the closed-patch (Buehler) test which is accepted in the United States.

Magnusson Maximization Test-Dermal/Intradermal Method

➤ *Procedure*

- Healthy, albino, Hartley guinea pigs weighing 300 to 500 grams are used. Older, larger guinea pigs are less sensitizable.

- Females, nulliparous and nonpregnant, are usually used because of their more tractable nature, however, males may be used.

- Generally, 10 to 25 animals per compound are used.

- Weigh the guinea pigs at the beginning of the study.

- Antigen with and without adjuvant is injected intradermally (see previous description in this chapter). Skin should be shaved and properly prepared before injection.

- Two rows of three injections are made, one on each side of the midline, one with 0.1 mL adjuvant only, one with 0.1 mL of test compound only, and the third with 0.1 mL test compound plus complete adjuvant.

- One week after intradermal injection, the area is again clipped and shaved.

- If the test compound is nonirritating, the skin is prepared with 10% sodium lauryl sulfate (SLS) in petrolatum 24 hours before patch is applied. The SLS is massaged into the skin with a glass rod. The SLS is used to induce a mild inflammatory response.

- The test compound in petrolatum is spread over a 2 × 4 cm patch of filter paper, in a thick, even layer.

- The patch is placed on the guinea pig's back and covered by overlapping impermeable, plastic tape.

- The patch is then secured by elastic bandage around the animal's torso.

- The bandage is left in place for 48 hours.

- Two weeks after topical application, the guinea pigs are treated with another topical application.

- Hair is removed from a 5 × 5 cm area of the flank by clipping and shaving.

- Test compound is applied to a 2 × 2 cm piece of filter paper as before.

- The patch is applied to the flank area and sealed as before for 24 hours.

- The treatment site is evaluated 24 hours after removal of the patch. This allows irritation due to the plastic tape sufficient time to subside.

- The test area is shaved three hours before being evaluated.

- The test area is evaluated again in another 24 hours.

- Redness represents a mild reaction. If uncertain about the mild reaction, repeat the treatment step in three to four days.

- Strongly sensitized animals display severe swelling and redness. Scores can be recorded using a four point scale, where 0 = no reaction, 1 = scattered mild redness, 2 = moderate and diffuse swelling, and 3 = intense redness and swelling.

- Histopathology of the skin will help differentiate mild irritation from a mild sensitivity reaction.

- Weigh the animals at the end of the study.

- A written report should be made containing the following information: name and description of the method used, species and strain used, positive control used, number and sex of animals used, beginning and ending weights of the animals, description of the grading system, and a summary in tabular form of each reading made on each animal.[193]

Buehler Closed-Patch Sensitization Test

This test is an irritancy screening test for various dilutions of compounds, usually 25%, 50%, 75% weight/volume, and undiluted concentrations are tested.

➤ *Procedure*

- The backs of healthy, albino guinea pigs are prepared by clipping the hair and scrubbing the skin.

- The diluted and undiluted compounds are applied to the previously prepared skin as a patch and the animal wrapped with an occlusive bandage (see Magnusson Method).

- The bandage is left for six (6) hours and then removed.

- The skin is washed with warm water and patted dry.

- Compound is applied to the same area (same concentration) once a week for three consecutive weeks.

- The skin is evaluated and scored at 24 and 48 hours, with 0 = no reaction, 1 = faint erythema, 2 = moderate erythema, and 3 = strong erythema with or without edema.

- The mildly irritating dose and the highest nonirritating dose are identified. These are used for the definitive study.

- Five to ten guinea pigs are prepared, clipped and scrubbed.

- The mildly irritating dose of the compound is applied to the skin, using the patch and occlusive bandage method, once a week for three consecutive weeks.

- Application of the compound should be to the same area of skin each week, unless the skin becomes severely irritated.

- Two weeks after the last dose, the highest nonirritating concentration is applied to the same areas of the skin on the back as a challenge dose.

- The skin is evaluated and scored, Buehler scores given above, 24 and 48 hours after the challenge dose was applied to the skin.

- Compounds that produce inconclusive results, should be retested at a higher compound concentration one to two weeks after the challenge dose was given.

Guinea Pig Antigenicity (Anaphylaxis) Test

➤ *Procedure*

- Guinea pigs are an established model for the study of immediate hypersensitivity reactions (anaphylaxis), responding to antigens with constriction of bronchial and bronchiolar smooth muscles. Sensitized guinea pigs exposed to an antigen may exhibit cyanosis, collapse, and death.

- Many dosing schedules and methods have been used for antigenicity testing, but all include sensitizing the guinea pig to a compound and administration of a challenge exposure to elicit a reaction.

- A common sensitization schedule entails giving animals a subcutaneous dose of compound once a week for three consecutive weeks. Test groups of animals are injected with test compound alone, test compound plus FCA, FCA alone, or saline, as a negative control.

- On day 31, from first sensitizing dose, the guinea pigs are administered the compound intravenously (IV), by aerosol, or by another route and the animals observed for signs of anaphlaxis, such as scratching, coughing, labored breathing, wretching, cyanosis, etc.

- Animals are monitored for 15 minutes and the response is scored, with 0 = no reaction to 5 = moribund, near death, or dead.

Sereny Test

The Sereny Test in guinea pigs is used to determine the virulence of *Shigella* strains and to screen different strains for vaccine efficacy. Bacteria is placed on the conjunctiva and cornea and the development of keratoconjunctivitis is monitored.[198]

necropsy

At the end of many studies it is necessary to examine the guinea pig after it has been euthanized. The animal's body, organs, and tissues are closely examined, and frequently collected for later microscopic examination. A complete guide to the necropsy of rodents has been published elsewhere.[199]

Equipment needed for a proper post-mortem examination includes:

- Disposable gloves, lab coat, protective eyewear, such as face mask, eye goggles, or safety glasses.

- A small metric ruler.

- Toothed and serrated tissue forceps.

- Scalpel blades and handles.

- Dissecting and small surgery scissors.

- A probe.

- Bone cutting forceps.

- Sterile swabs for bacteriologic culture.

- Assorted needles and syringes.

- Saline for washing samples and paper towels for absorption of fluids.

- Specimen containers.

- 10% neutral buffered formalin or other fixative.

Note: Necropsy equipment will need to be resharpened periodically.

The necropsy should be performed within a dedicated necropsy room or in a designated necropsy area that can be easily cleaned and sanitized. Stainless steel surfaces are best, along with downdraft ventilation. If this is unavailable, then a designated area, preferably with a fume hood, away from animals, feed, bedding, and personnel may be used.

Buffered formalin is the most commonly used fixative. It may be made from formaldehyde or purchased commercially already prepared. It should be stored in airtight containers and within a fume hood, if possible. Many people exhibit ocular and respiratory allergic reactions to formaldehyde. Also, formaldehyde is considered a human carcinogen.[200] For these reasons, formalin fixatives should be used and stored with caution.

Appropriate personal protective equipment should be worn by anyone performing a guinea pig necropsy. This should include a labcoat, gloves, and a face mask or protective eyeglasses or goggles. Care should be taken to minimize the chance of infection with zoonotic agents. However, the chance of this is slight when purpose-bred guinea pigs from a reputable vendor have been used.

A consistent necropsy technique should be developed by all persons routinely performing guinea pig necropsies. It should follow a set pattern each time an animal is examined. The best results can be obtained from an animal that has recently been euthanized. Severe postmortem changes will occur if an animal is left at room temperature or warmer for a short period of time. Freezing of the guinea pig's body will also induce numerous postmortem artifacts.

➤ *Method*

1. Record the guinea pig's identification number.

2. Weigh the guinea pig.

3. Perform an in-depth external examination including sex of the animal; general body condition; fur condition; obvious wounds or abnormalities; discharge from mouth, eyes, ears, nose; and urine or fecal staining of the fur.

4. Blood may need to be collected for serologic evaluation in some cases before the guinea pig is euthanized

5. Place the animal on its back on an appropriate surface.

6. Wet the fur with alcohol to keep the fur from falling into the animal. Be very careful of flaming instruments for sterile tissue collection. The alcohol soaked guinea pig will catch on fire if instruments are not cooled first.

7. Make a superficial midline incision from the jaw to the scrotum or vulva.

8. Carefully incise and retract the skin on both sides.

9. Dissect through the muscle in the neck to observe the salivary, thymus, thyroid, and parathyroid glands

10. Carefully incise the abdominal wall.

11. Cut the ribs on each side of the chest, incise the diaphragm, and reflect this area.

12. Carefully examine all organs *in situ.* Examine all surfaces for spots, discoloration, or any other abnormality. Examine the inner surface of the thoracic and abdominal cavities. Collect, culture, and cytologically examine any abnormal fluid found within the body cavities.

13. Remove the heart, lungs, and trachea by cutting the trachea, holding it with the forceps with light traction, and cutting all attachments to the thorax and diaphragm. Thoroughly examine these organs.

14. Collect culture swabs of abnormalities that appear to be of bacterial origin.

15. Collect all abnormal tissues and masses and place in 10% buffered formalin for later histopathologic evaluation.

16. Clean and disinfect all equipment and surfaces.

resources

Examples of vendors and organizations are included in this chapter to provide users of this book with information regarding literature sources, guinea pigs, caging, and materials. The lists are not exhaustive nor meant to imply endorsement of one vendor over another, but are meant to be used as a starting point for developing a database of resources.

organizations

Many professional organizations exist which can provide initial contacts for obtaining information regarding specific issues related to the care and use of laboratory animals. Membership in these organizations allows the laboratory animal science professional to stay abreast of changing regulatory guidelines, improvements in methodology and procedures, and current animal health issues. Relevant organizations are described here.

American Association for Laboratory Animal Science (AALAS). 70 Timber Creek Drive, Cordova, TN 38018 (Tel: 901-754-8620 and Fax On Demand: 901-754-2546). AALAS serves a diverse professional group. Members range from principal investigators to animal caretakers to veterinarians. Two journals, *Contemporary Topics in Laboratory Animal Science* and

Laboratory Animal Science are published by AALAS, and serve as the primary means of communicating relevant information within the organization. AALAS sponsors a program for certification of laboratory animal science professionals at three levels: assistant laboratory animal technician (ALAT), laboratory animal technician (LAT), and laboratory animal technologist (LATG). The AALAS-affiliated Institute for Laboratory Animal Management (ILAM) is a program designed to provide state of the art training in laboratory animal facility management. In addition, the association sponsors an annual meeting. Many areas of the country have active local branches, with regular meetings, professional seminars, and smaller regional meetings.

Association for Assessment and Accreditation of Laboratory Animal Care International, Inc. Executive Director, 11300 Rockville Pike, Suite 1211, Rockville, Maryland 20852-3035 (Tel: 301-231-5353). AAALAC International is a nonprofit organization which provides a mechanism for peer evaluation of laboratory animal care programs. Since its formation in 1965, AAALAC accreditation has become widely accepted as strong evidence of a quality research animal care and use program. Application for accreditation and site-visit reports are reviewed using the *Guide for the Care and Use of Laboratory Animals* published by the Institute of Laboratory Animal Resources as a guideline.

American College of Laboratory Animal Medicine (ACLAM). Executive Director (current: Dr. Charles McPherson, 200 Summerwinds Drive, Cary, North Carolina 27511). The college is recognized by the American Veterinary Medical Association as a specialty of veterinary medicine, and board certifies veterinarians as Diplomates in laboratory animal medicine by means of rigorous examination, experience, and publication requirements. The group encourages education, training, and research in laboratory animal medicine through activities such as the annual ACLAM forum and sessions at the annual AALAS meeting.

American Society of Laboratory Animal Practitioners (ASLAP). This association has a membership consisting of veterinarians engaged in some aspect of laboratory animal medicine.

The society publishes a newsletter to foster communication between members and sponsors annual meetings, generally in conjunction with annual meetings of AALAS or the American Veterinary Medical Association. Current contact information may be obtained through AALAS.

Laboratory Animal Management Association (LAMA). P.O. Box 1744, Silver Springs, MD 20915. This organization serves as a mechanism for information exchange between individuals with management responsibility for laboratory animal facilities. The group publishes the *LAMA Review* and sponsors periodic meetings. Contacts change annually with the elected leadership, but current contact information is available from AALAS.

International Council for Laboratory Animal Science (ICLAS). Current contact: Professor Osmo Hanninen, Secretary General, Dept. of Physiology, University of Kuopio, P.O. Box 1627, Kuopio, Finland. The aim of ICLAS is to promote and coordinate the development of laboratory animal science throughout the world, including international collaborations of laboratory animal scientists, humane animal care and use of research animals, and the monitoring of quality in research animals worldwide. The organization sponsors programs in microbiological and genetic monitoring of research animals and assists developing countries in pursuing their objectives in improving the care and use of laboratory animals. Membership consists of national members, scientific members, and scientific union members.

Institute for Laboratory Animal Resources (ILAR). 2101 Constitution Avenue NW, Washington, D.C. 20418 (Tel: 202-334-2590). The institute functions under the auspices of the National Research Council to develop and make available scientific and technical information on laboratory animals and other biological resources. ILAR promotes high-quality, humane care of animals, and the appropriate use of animals and alternatives. A number of publications are available from ILAR, including the *Guide for the Care and Use of Laboratory Animals* and the *ILAR Journal.*

publications

A number of published materials, books, and periodicals are valuable as additional reference materials.

Books

1. *The Biology of the Guinea Pig,* edited by P.J. Manning and J. E. Wagner, 1976. Academic Press, Inc., 111 Fifth Avenue, New York, NY 10003.

2. *The Biology and Medicine of Rabbits and Rodents,* by J. E. Harkness and J. E. Wagner, 1995. Williams and Wilkins, Baltimore, MD 21298-9724.

3. *Formulary for Laboratory Animals,* by C.T. Hawk and S. L. Leary, 1995. Iowa State University Press, Ames, IA 50014.

4. *Laboratory Animal Anesthesia,* by P.A. Flecknell, 1987. Academic Press, Inc. 525 B. Street, Suite 1900, San Diego, CA 92101.

5. *Handbook of Veterinary Anesthesia,* by W. W. Muir, J.A.E. Hubell, R.T. Skarda, and R. M. Bedarski, 1995. C.V. Mosby Co., 11830 Westline Industrial Drive, St. Louis, MO 63146.

6. *Necropsy Guide: Rodents and the Rabbit,* by D. B. Feldman and J. C. Seely, 1988. CRC Press, Inc., 2000 Corporate Blvd. N. W., Boca Raton, FL 33431.

Periodicals

1. *Laboratory Animal Science.* Published by the American Association for Laboratory Animal Science. For contact information, see above listing for AALAS.

2. *Contemporary Topics in Laboratory Animal Science.* Published by the American Association for Laboratory Animal Science. For contact information, see above listing for AALAS.

3. *Laboratory Animals.* Published by the Royal Society of Medicine Press, 1 Wimpole Street, London WIM 8AE, UK.

4. *Lab Animal.* Published by Nature Publishing Co. 345 Park Avenue South, New York, NY 10010-1707.

5. *ILAR Journal.* Published by the Institute of Laboratory Animal Resources, National Research Council. For contact information, see above listing for ILAR.

electronic resources

Many online sources of information relevant to the care and use of laboratory animals, including guinea pigs, are available. These include the following:

1. **ALPHA.** This site includes American Association for Laboratory Animal Science information services, file transfer protocol libraries, current information in laboratory animal science, and connections to other pertinent web sites. The system originates from the American Association for Laboratory Animal Science (American Association for Laboratory Animal Science). Some portions of the system are open to the general public and may be accessed at **http://www.aalas.org** or **http://205.231.134.98**

2. **Comparative Medicine Discussion List (COMPMED).** An electronic mailing list available through the internet, COMPMED is a valuable means to quickly tap into the expertise of laboratory animal science professionals around the world. At the time of publication, those interested in using this resource should subscribe to **listserv@wuvmd.wustl.edu** and mail to **compmed @wuvmd.wustl.edu.**

3. **Network of Animal Health (NOAH).** NOAH is a commercial online service sponsored by the American Veterinary Medical Association. A number of forums cover a variety of topics, some of which would be of interest to those charged with the care and use of laboratory guinea pigs. Additional information can be obtained from the American Veterinary Medical Association, 1931 N. Meachum Road, Suite 100, Schaumburg, Il; 1-800-248-2862; e-mail: 72662.345@compuserv.com

4. **The NETVET.** The netvet is a collection of world wide web pages and links covering every aspect of veterinary medicine. Animal vendors, research institutions, scientific organizations, along with electronic versions of laws, regulations, and policies are found among its many links. Dr. Ken Boschert of Washington University is the site manager and its originator. The Netvet can be accessed at **http://netvet.wustl.edu/.**

animal sources

Guinea pigs are commercially available from a large number of suppliers. These vendors vary widely in size and quality. The purchase of specific pathogen-free (SPF) animals is strongly encouraged, and is often required in large facilities where inadvertent admission of an infectious agent would threaten other animals or studies. Vendors should be asked in advance of purchase for documentation regarding the health status of their guinea pig colony. A veterinarian or knowledgeable animal facility manager can provide assistance if needed with interpretation of the documentation. While it is impractical to list all vendors here, the following are some examples of vendors which supply guinea pigs.

1. Ace Animals, Inc., P.O. Box 155, 2025 Ridge Road, Boyertown, PA 19512 (Tel: 610-367-6047).

2. Camm Research Lab Animals, 414 Black Oak Ridge Road, Wayne, NJ 07470 (Tel: 201-694-0703).

3. Charles River Laboratories, 251 Ballardvale Street, Wilmington, MA 01887 (Tel: 508-658-6000).

4. Davidson's Mill Breeding Laboratories, 231 Fresh Pond Road, Jamesburg, NJ 08831 (Tel: 908-821-9094).

5. Elm Hill Breeding Laboratories, Inc., 71 Elm Street, Chelmsford, MA 01824 (Tel: 508-256-2545).

6. HRP, Inc., P.O. Box 7200, Denver, PA 17517-0200 (Tel:1-800-345-4114).

7. Harlan Sprague Dawley, Inc., P.O. Box 29176, Indianapolis, In 46229-0176 (Tel: 317-894-7521).

8. Hilltop Lab Animals, P.O. Box 183, RD #1, Hilltop, Scottdale, PA 15683 (Tel: 412-887-8480).

9. Simonsen Laboratories, Inc., 1180-C Day Road, Gilroy, CA 95020-9308 (Tel: 408-847-2002).

feed

Although small local suppliers can often provide high-quality feed to research facilities, it is more frequently obtained from large vendors such as those listed below. Because of the unique dietary requirements of guinea pigs (vitamin C), selection of the vendor, distributor, and shipping and holding facilities must be carefully considered.

1. Bio-Serv, Inc., P.O. Box 450, 8th and Harrison Streets, Frenchtown, NJ 08825 (Tel: 1-800-473-2155).

2. Harlan Teklad, Inc., P.O. Box 44220, Madison, WI 53744-4220 (Tel: 1-800-483-5523).

3. PMI/Purina Mills, Inc., 505 North 4th Street, P. O. Box 548, Richmond, IN 47375 (Tel: 1-800-227-8941).

equipment

Equipment needs are different for each laboratory and experimental protocol. Caging, watering devices, feeders, sanitation supplies, restrainers, anesthesia equipment, and specific research devices (i.e., osmotic pumps) are examples of the many products available to assist the researcher in working with animals humanely and efficiently. Items are available from multiple sources, of which a number are listed. Cages must meet the requirements specified by relevant regulatory agencies, as well as fitting the housing standards in each facility. Pharmaceutical items should only be ordered and used under the direction of a licensed veterinarian.

Possible Sources of Cages and Research and Veterinary Supplies

Item	Source
Cages and supplies	4, 5, 11, 14, 21, 22, 23, 25, 28
Veterinary and surgical supplies	1, 12, 17, 18, 19, 30
Gas anesthesia equipment	1, 17, 19, 25, 29, 30
Restrainers	3, 4, 7, 8, 16, 17, 20, 21, 26
Cervical collars	24, 30
Sanitation and disinfection	10, 13, 27
Syringes and needles	1, 8, 12, 16, 18, 19
Osmotic pumps	6, 17, 30
Necropsy tools	8, 16, 30
Electrophysiology equipment	15, 17, 30
Animal identification supplies	1, 2, 7, 9, 17
Cage washer repair	31

contact information for sources

1. A. J. Buck & Sons Inc., 11407 Cronhill Drive, Owing Mills, MD 21117 (Tel: 1-800-638-8672).

2. AVID, 3179 Hammer Avenue, Norco, CA 91670 (Tel: 1-800-336-2843).

3. Alice King Chatham Medical Arts, 11915-17 Inglewood Avenue, Hawthorne, CA 90250 (Tel: 310-970-1063).

4. Allentown Caging Equipment, Inc., Route 526, P.O. Box 698, Allentown, NJ 08501-0698 (Tel: 609-259-7051).

5. Alternative Design Manufacturing and Supply, 16396 Old Highway 68, Siloam Springs, AR 72761 (Tel: 1-800-320-2459).

6. Alza Corporation, 950 Page Mill Road, P.O. Box 10950, Palo Alto, CA 94303-0802 (Tel: 1-800-692-2990).

7. Ancare Corp., 2647 Grand Avenue, P.O. Box 814, Bellmore, NY 11710-0814 (Tel: 1-800-645-6379).

8. Baxter Diagnostics, Inc., Scientific Products Division, 1430 Waukegan Road, McGaw Park, Il 60085-9988 (Tel: 1-800-964-5227).

9. BioMedic Data Systems, Inc., 255 W. Spring Valley Avenue, Marywood, NJ 07607 (Tel: 1-800-526-BMDS).

10. Biosentry, Inc., 1481 Rock Mountain Boulevard, Stone Mountain, GA 30083-9986 (Tel: 1-800-788-4246).

11. Britz-Heidbrink, Inc. P.O. Box 1179, Wheatland, WY 82201-1179 (Tel: 307-322-4040).

12. Butler Co., Inc., 5000 Brandenton Avenue, Dublin, OH 43017 (Tel: 1-800-225-7911).

13. Convatec, Calgon Vestal Contamination Control, P.O. Box 147, St. Louis, MO 63166-0147, (Tel: 1-800-325-0966).

14. Fenco Cage Products, 1188 Dorchester Avenue, Dorchester, MA 02125-1503 (Tel: 1-800-233-2243).

15. Fine Science Tools, Inc., 373-G Vintage Park Drive, Foster City, CA 94404 (Tel: 1-800-521-2109).

16. Fisher Scientific, Inc., 711 Forbes Avenue, Pittsburgh, PA 15219-4785 (Tel: 1-800-766-7000).

17. Harvard Apparatus, Inc., 22 Pleasant Street, South Natick, MA 01760 (Tel: 1-800-272-2775).

18. IDE Interstate, Inc., 1500 New Horizons Boulevard, Amityville, NY 11701 (Tel: 1-800-666-8100).

19. J. A. Webster, Inc., 86 Leominster Road, Sterling, MA 01564 (Tel: 1-800-225-7911).

20. K.L.A.S.S., Inc., 4960 Aladen Expressway, Suite 233, San Jose, CA 95118 (Tel: 408-266-1235).

21. Lab Products, Inc., 255 West Spring Valley Avenue, P.O. Box 808, Maywood, NJ 07607 (Tel: 1-800-526-0469).

22. Lenderking Caging Products, Inc., 1000 South Linwood Avenue, Baltimore, MD 21224 (Tel: 410-276-2237).

23. Lock Solutions, Inc., P.O. Box 611, Kenilworth, NJ 07033 (Tel: 1-800-947-0304).

24. Lomir Biomedical, Inc., 99 East Main Street, Malone, NY 12953 (Tel: 518-483-7697).

25. Otto Environmental, 6914 North 124th Street, Milwaukee, WI 53224 (Tel: 1-800-484-5363, Ext. 6886).

26. P.A.M., Inc., 47 North Front Street, Souderton, PA 18964 (Tel: 1-800-237-3373).

27. Rochester Midland, Inc., 333 Hollenbeck Street, P.O. Box 1515, Rochester, NY 14603-1515 (Tel: 1-800-836-1627).

28. Suburban Surgical Company, Inc., 275 Twelfth Street, Wheeling, IL 60090 (Tel: 1-800-323-7366).

29. Vetamac. Inc., P. O. Box 178, Rossville, IN 46065 (Tel: 1-800-334-1583).

30. Viking Products, Inc., P.O. Box 2142, Medford Lakes, NJ 08055 (Tel: 1-800-920-1033).

31. Washers International, Ltd., 231 Dellwood Road, Amherst, NY 13226 (Tel: 1-716-836-2977).

commercial laboratories for animal health monitoring

1. Charles River Laboratories, 251 Ballardvale Street, Wilmington, MA 01887 (Tel: 1-800-522-7287).

2. Microbiological Associates, 9900 Blackwell Road, Rockville, MD 20850 (Tel: 1-800-756-5658).

3. University of Miami, Division of Comparative Pathology, Pathology Reference Services, P. O. Box 016960 (R-5),Miami, FL 33101 (Tel: 1-800-596-7390).

4. University of Missouri — Columbia, Research Animal Diagnostic and Investigative Laboratory, 1600 East Rollins Road, Columbia, MO 65211 (Tel: 1-800-669-0825).

bibliography

1. Weir, B. J., Notes on the origin of the domestic guinea pig, in *Symposia of the Zoological Society of London,* No. 34, Rowlands, I. W., and Weir, B. J., Eds., Academic Press, London, 1974, 437.

2. *Annual Report to Congress on Animal Welfare Enforcement,* United States Department of Agriculture, 1994.

3. Lane-Petter, W. and Porter, G., in *Animals for Research,* Lane-Petter, W. Ed., Academic Press, New York, 1963, 287.

4. DeWeck, D. L. and Festing, F. M. W., Investigations for which the guinea pig is well suited, in *Inbred and Genetically Defined Strains of Laboratory Animals,* Altman, P.L., and Katz, D. D. Eds., Fed. Am. Soc. Exp. Biol., Bethesda, Maryland, 1979, 507.

5. Festing, M. F. W., The guinea-pig, in *The UFAW Handbook on the Care and Management of Laboratory Animals,* Hume, C.W. Ed., Churchill Livingstone, Edinburgh, 1976, 229.

6. Wagner, J. E., Introduction and Taxonomy, in *The Biology of the Guinea Pig,* Wagner, J. E. and Manning, P.J. Eds., Academic Press, New York, 1976, 1.

7. Simpson, G. G., The principles of classification and classification of mammals, *Bulletin of the American Museum of Natural History,* 85, 1945, 93.

8. D'Erchia, A. M., Gissi, C., Pesole, G., Saccone, C., and Arnason, U., The guinea pig is not a rodent, *Nature,* 381, 597, 1996.

9. King, J.A., Social relationships of the domestic guinea pig living under semi-natural conditions, *Ecology,* 37, 221, 1956.

10. Rood, J. P., Ecological and behavioral comparisons of three genera of Argentine cavies, *Animal Behavior Monographs,* 5, 1, 1972.

11. Shevach, E. M., Festing, M. F., and deWeck, A. L., Inbred and partially inbred strain: guinea pig, in *Inbred and Genetically Defined Strains of Laboratory Animals,* Altman, P.L. and Katz, D. D. Eds., Fed. Am. Soc. Exp. Biol, Bethesda, Maryland, 1979, 507.

12. Reed, C. and O'Donoghue, J. L., A new guinea pig mutant with abnormal hair production and immunodeficiency, *Laboratory Animal Science,* 29, 744, 1979.

13. Festing, M. F. W., Genetics, in *The Biology of the Guinea Pig,* Wagner, J. E., and Manning, P. J., Eds., Academic Press, New York, 1976, 99.

14. Nicholls, E. E., A study of the spontaneous activity of the guinea pig, *Journal of Comparative Psychology,* 2, 303, 1922.

15. Grant, E. C. and Macintosh, J. H., A comparison of the social postures of some common laboratory rodents, *Behavior,* 21, 246, 1963.

16. Berryman, J., Guinea pig vocalizations, *Guinea Pig Newsletter,* 2, 9, 1970.

17. Berryman, J. C., Guinea pig responses to conspecific vocalizations: Playback experiments, *Behavioral and Neural Biology,* 31, 476, 1981.

18. Beach, F. A., Ontogeny of "coitus-related" reflexes in the female guinea pig, *Proceedings of the National Academy of Science — U.S.*, 56, 526 1966.

19. Cooper, G. and Schiller, A. L., *Anatomy of the Guinea Pig*, Harvard University Press, Cambridge Massachusettes, 1975.

20. Breazile, J. E. and Brown, E. M., Anatomy, in *The Biology of the Guinea Pig*, Wagner, J. E., and Manning, P.J. Eds., Academic Press, New York, 1976, 53.

21. Harkness, J. E. and Wagner, J. E., Biology and husbandry, *The Biology and Medicine of Rabbits and Rodents*, Lea & Febiger, Philadelphia, 1989, 19.

22. Charles River Technical Bulletin, Charles River Laboratories, Wilmington, Massachusettes, 1, 1, 1982.

23. Hong, C. C., Ediger, R. D., Raetz, R., and Djurickovic, S., Measurement of guinea pig body surface area, *Laboratory Animal Science*, 27, 474, 1977.

24. Herrington, L. P., The heat regulation of small laboratory animals at various environmental temperatures, *American Journal of Physiology*, 129, 123, 1940.

25. Jilge, B., The gastrointestinal transit time in the guinea-pig, *Zeitschrift fur Versuchstierkunde*, 22, 204, 1980.

26. Navia, J. M. and Hunt, C. E., Nutrition, nutritional diseases, and nutritional research applications, in *The Biology of the Guinea Pig*, Wagner, J. E. and Manning, P.J. Eds., Academic Press, New York, 1976, 235.

27. Zeman, F. J. and Wilbur, C. G., Hematology in the normal male guinea pig, *Life Science*, 4, 871, 1965.

28. Bunn, H. F., Differences in the interaction of 2,3-diphosphoglycerate with certain mammalian hemoglobins, *Science*, 172, 1049, 1971.

29. Bethlenfalvay, N. C., Cytologic demonstration of methemoglobin and carboxyhemoglobin in certain vertebrates, *American Journal of Veterinary Research*, 33, 1017, 1972.

30. Ernstrom, U. and Sandberg, G., On the origin of Foa-Kurloff cells, *Scandinavian Journal of Haematology*, 8, 380, 1971.

31. Dean, M. F. and Muir, H., The characterization of a protein-polysaccharide isolated from Kurloff cells of the guinea pig, *Biochemistry Journal*, 118, 783, 1970.

32. Revell, P. A., Vernon-Roberts, B., and Gray, A., The distribution and ultrastructure of the Kurloff cell in the guinea pig, *Journal of Anatomy*, 109, 187, 1971.

33. Marshall, A. H. E., Swettenham, K. V., Vernon-Roberts, B., and Revell, P. A., Studies on the function of the Kurloff cell, *International Archive of Allergy and Applied Immunology*, 40, 137, 1971.

34. Ernstrom, U., Hormonal influences on thymic release of lymphocytes into the blood, *Ciba Foundation Study Group*, 36, 53, 1970.

35. Calman, H. N., Corticosteroids and lymphoid cells, *New England Journal of Medicine*, 287, 388, 1972.

36. Ernstrom, U. and Larsson, B., Determination of thymic blood flow in guinea-pigs of different ages, *Acta Pathologica et Microbiologica Scandinavica Section A*, 78, 366, 1970.

37. Kaspareit, J., Messow, C., and Edel, J., Blood coagulation studies in guinea pigs *(Cavia porcellus)*, *Laboratory Animals*, 22, 206, 1988.

38. Mills, D. C. B., Platelet aggregation and platelet nucleotide concentration in different species, *Symposium of the Zoological Society of London*, 27, 99, 1970.

39. Altman, P. L. and Dittmer, D. S., Eds., *The Biology Data Book*, Federation of American Societies for Experimental Biology, Bethesda, 1974.

40. Lucarelli, G. and Butturini, U., The control of foetal and neonatal erythropoiesis, *Proceedings of the Royal Society of Medicine*, 60, 1036, 1967.

41. Griffiths, D. A. and Rieke, W. O., A comparison of quanitative hematological values in two strains of normal guinea pigs, *Experimental Hematology*, 18, 36, 1969.

42. Scarborough, R. H., The blood picture of normal laboratory animals, *Yale Journal of Biology and Medicine*, 3, 169, 1931.

43. Banerjee, V., Relative variation in some vertebrate erythrocytes, *Naturwissenschaften*, 53, 233, 1966.

44. Edmonson, P. W. and Wyburn, J. R., The erythrocyte lifespan, red cell mass and plasma volume of normal guinea pigs as determined by the use of [51]chromium, [32]phosphorous labelled di-iso-propyl fluorophosphonate and [131]iodine labelled human serum albumin, *British Journal of Experimental Pathology*, 44, 72, 1963.

45. Constable, B. J., Changes in blood volume and blood picture during the life of the rat and guinea-pig from birth to maturity, *Journal of Physiology*, 167, 229, 1963.

46. Payne, B. J., Lewis, H. B., Murchison, T. E., and Hart, E. A., Hematology of laboratory animals, in *Handbook of Laboratory Animal Science Vol. III*, Melby, E. C., and Altman, N. H., Eds., CRC Press, Cleveland, Ohio, 1976, 383.

47. Innes, J., Innes, E. M., and Moore, C. V., The hematologic changes induced in guinea pigs by the prolonged administration of pteroyl glutamic acid antagonists, *Journal of Laboratory Clinical Medicine*, 34, 883, 1949.

48. Bilbey, D. L. J. and Nichol, T., Normal blood picture of the guinea pig, *Nature (London)*, 176, 1218, 1955.

49. Hurt, J. P. and Krigman, M. R., Selected procoagulants in the guinea pig, *American Journal of Physiology*, 218, 832, 1970.

50. Warner, E. D., Brinkhous, K. M., and Smith, H. P., Plasma prothrombin levels in various vertebrates, *American Journal of Physiology*, 125, 296, 1939.

51. Hwang, S. W. and Wosilait, W. D., Comparative and developmental studies on blood coagulation, *Comparative Biochemical Physiology*, 37, 595, 1970.

52. Sisk, D. B., Physiology, in *The Biology of the Guinea Pig*, Wagner, J. E., and Manning, P. J. Eds., Academic Press, New York, 1976, 53.

53. Laird, C. W., Biochemical constituents of serum, in *Handbook of Laboratory Animal Science Vol. III,* Melby, E. C., and Altman, N. H., Eds., CRC Press, Cleveland, Ohio, 1974, 365.

54. Anderson, R. R., Nixon, D. A., and Akasha, M. A., Total and free thyroxine and triiodothyronine in blood serum of animals, *Comparative Biochemistry and Physiology,* 89, 401, 1988.

55. Petelenz, T., Electrocardiogram of the guinea pig, *Acta Physiologica Polonica,* 22, 113, 1971.

56. Pratt, C. G. L., The electrocardiogram of the guinea pig, *Journal of Physiology (London),* 92, 268, 1938.

57. Mikiskova, H. and Mikiska, A., Some elctrophysiologic methods for studying the action of narcotic agents in animals, with special reference to industrial solvents: a review, *British Journal of Industrial Medicine,* 25, 81, 1968.

58. Fara, J. W. and Catlett, R. H., Cardiac response and social behavior in the guinea-pig (*Cavia porcellus), Animal Behavior,* 19, 514, 1971.

59. Marshall, L.H. and Hanna, C. H., Direct measurement of arterial blood pressure in the guinea pig, *Proceeding for the Society of Experimental Biology and Medicine,* 92, 31, 1956.

60. Guyton, A. C., Measurement of the respiratory volumes of laboratory animals, *American Journal of Physiology,* 150, 70, 1947.

61. Siaud, P., Denoroy, L., Assenmacher, I. and Alonso, G., Comparative immunocutochemical study of the catecholaminergic and peptide afferenent innervation to the doral vagal complex in rat and guinea pig, *Journal of Comparative Neurology,* 290, 323, 1989.

62. De Schaepdrijver, L., Simoens, P., Lauwers, H., and De Geest, J. P., Retinal vascular patterns in domestic animals, *Research in Veterinary Science,* 47, 34, 1989.

63. Keller, E., Kohl, J., and Kollers, E. A., Location of pulmonary stretch receptors in the guinea pig, *Respiratory Physiology,* 76, 149, 1989.

64. Freund, M., Initiation and development of semen production in the guinea pig, *Fertility and Sterility*, 13, 190, 1962.

65. Hill, P. M. M. and Young, M., Use of the guinea-pig foetal placenta, perfused *in situ*, as a model to study the placental transfer of pharmacological substances, *British Journal of Pharmacology*, 47, 655, 1973.

66. Mill, P. G. and Reed, M., The onset of first oestrus in the guinea-pig and the effects of gonadotropins and oestradiol in the immature animal, *Journal of Endocrinology*, 50, 329, 1971.

67. Stockard, C. R. and Papanicolaou, G. N., The existence of a typical oestrous cycle in the guinea-pig-with a study of its histological and physiological changes, *American Journal of Anatomy*, 22, 225, 1917.

68. Boling, J. L., Blandau, R. J., Wilson, J. G., and Young, W. C., Post-parutitional heat response newborn and adult guinea pigs. Data on parturition, *Proceedings for the Society of Experimental Biology and Medicine*, 42, 128, 1939.

69. McKeown, T. and MacMahon, B., The influence of litter size and litter order on length of gestation and early postnatal growth in the guinea-pig, *Journal of Endocrinology*, 13, 195, 1956.

70. Bruce, H. M. and Parks, A. S., Feeding and breeding of laboratory animals, *Journal of Hygiene*, 46, 434, 1948.

71. Mepham, T. B. and Beck, N. F. G., Variation in the yield and composition of milk throughout lactation in the guinea pig (*Cavia porcellus*), *Comparative Biochemistry and Physiology A*, 45, 273, 1973.

72. Young, W. C., Dempsey, E. W., and Myers, H. I., Cyclic reproductive behavior in the female guinea pig, *Journal of Comparative Physiology and Psychology*, 19, 313, 1935.

73. Ford, D.H. and Young, W. C., Duration of the first cyclic vaginal openings in maturing guinea pigs and related ovarian conditions, *Anatomical Record*, 115, 495, 1953.

74. Reed, M., and Hounslow, W. F., Induction of ovulation in the guinea-pig, *Journal of Endocrinology*, 49, 203, 1971.

75. Harned, M. A. and Casida, L. E., Failure to obtain group synchrony of estrus in the guinea pig, *Journal of Mammology*, 53, 223, 1972.

76. Stockard, C. R., and Papanicolaou, G. N., The vaginal closure membrane, copulation, and the vaginal plug in the guinea-pig, with further considerations of the oestrou rhythm, *Biology Bulletin*, 37, 222, 1919.

77. Herrick, E. H., The duration of pregnancy in guinea-pigs after removal and also after transplantation of the ovaries, *Anatomical Record*, 39, 193, 1928.

78. Hisaw, F. L., Zarrow, M. X., Money, W. L., Talmage, R. V. N., and Abramowitz, A. A., Importance of the female reproductive tract in the formation of relaxin, *Endocrinology*, 34, 122, 1944.

79. Linzell, J. L., The role of the mammary glands in reproduction, *Research in Reproduction*, 3, 2, 1971.

80. Breckenridge, W. C. and Kuksis, A., Molecular weight distributions of milk fat triglycerides from seven species, *Journal of Lipid Research*, 8, 473, 1967.

81. Nelson, W. L., Kaye, A., Moore, M., Williams, H. H., and Herrington, B. L., Milking techniques and composition of guinea pig milk, *Journal of Nutrition*, 44, 585, 1951.

82. Ruys, T., ed., Handbook of Facilities Planning, Volume 2 Laboratory Animal Facilities, Van Nostrand Reinhold, New York, 1991.

83. Committee on the Care and Use of Laboratory Animals of the Institute of Laboratory Animal Resources, *Guide for the Care and Use of Laboratory Animals*, National Academy Press, Washington, 1996.

84. CFR (Code of Federal Regulations), Title 9, Parts 1, 2, and 3 (Docket 89-130), Federal Register, 54 (168), August 31, 1989, and 9 CFR Part 3 (Docket 90-218), Federal Register, 56 (32), February 15, 1991.

85. Bailey, K. J., Stephens, D. B., and Delaney, C. E., Observations on the effects of vibration and noise on plasma ACTH and zinc levels, pregnancy and respiration rate in the guinea pig, *Laboratory Animals*, 20, 101, 1986.

86. Pye, A., Comparison of various short noise exposures in albino and pigmented guinea pigs, *Archives of Oto-Rhino-Laryngology*, 243, 411, 1987.

87. White, W. J., Balk, M. W., and Lang, C. M., Use of cage space by guinea pigs, *Laboratory Animals*, 23, 208, 1989.

88. Committee on Rodents of Institute of Laboratory Animal Resources, *Laboratory Animal Management — Rodents*, National Academy Press, Washington, 1996, 44.

89. Ediger, R. D., Care and management, in *The Biology of the Guinea Pig*, Wagner, J. E., and Manning, P.J. Eds., Academic Press, New York, 1976, 5.

90. DiGirolamo, M., Ander, B. L., and Francendese, A. A., Development and testing of an automated food dispenser for small rodents, *Laboratory Animal Science*, 31, 476, 1981.

91. Dunham, W. B., Young, M., and Tsao, C. S., Interferences by bedding materials in animal test systems involving ascorbic acid depletion, *Laboratory Animal Science*, 44, 283, 1994.

92. Plank, S. J. and Irwin, R., Infertility of guinea pigs on sawdust bedding, *Laboratory Animals*, 16, 9, 1966.

93. Marshal, L., Schutz, M., Bilsing, A., and Nichelmann, M., Preference for bedding material in growing guinea pigs (*Cavia porcellus*), *Experimental Animal Science*, 37, 109, 1994-1996.

94. van der Weerd, H. A. and Baumans, V, Environmental Enrichment in Rodents, in *Environmental Enrichment Information Resources for Laboratory Animals*, 1965-1995, AWIC Resource Series no. 2, 1996, 145.

95. Manning, P. J., Wagner, J. E., and Harkness, J. E., Biology and diseases of guinea pigs, in *Laboratory Animal Medicine*, J. G. Fox, B. J. Cohen, and F. M. Loew, eds., Academic Press, Orlando, 1984, 149.

96. Witt, W. M., Hubbard, G. B., and Fanton, J. W., Streptococcus pneumoniae arthritis and osteomyelitis with vitamin C. deficiency in guinea pigs, *Laboratory Animal Science*, 38, 192, 1988.

97. Ryan, L. J., Maina, C. V., Hopkins, R. K., and Carlow. C. K. S., Effectiveness of hand cleaning in sanitizing rabbit cages, *Contemporary Topics in Laboratory Animal Science*, 32, 21, 1992.

98. Wardrip, C. L., Artwohl, J. E., and Bennett, B. T., A review of the role of temperature vs. time in an effective cage sanitization program, *Contemporary Topics in Laboratory Animal Science*, 33, 66, 1994.

99. Animal Welfare Act, United States P.L. 89-544, 1966; P.L. 91-579, 1970; P.L. 94-279, 1976; and P.L. 99-198, 1985 (The Food Security Act).

100. Health Research Extension Act, United States P.L. 99-158, 1985.

101. Office of Protection from Research Risks, *Public Health Service Policy on Humane Care and Use of Laboratory Animals*, 1985.

102. CFR 21 (Food and Drugs), Part 58, Subparts A-K; CFR Title 40 (Protection of Environment), Part 160, Subparts A-J; CFR Title 40 (Protection of Environment), Part 792, Subparts A-L, 1978, 1995.

103. Bowman, P. J., A flexible occupational health and safety program for laboratory animal care and use programs, *Contemporary Topics in Laboratory Animal Science*, 30, 15, 1991.

104. Centers for Disease Control and National Institutes of Health (CDC/NIH), *Biosafety in Microbiological and Biomedical Laboratories*, NHS Pub. No. (NIH) 93-8395, CDC/NIH, Atlanta, 1993.

105. Laber-Laird, K. and Proctor, M., An example of a rodent health monitoring program, *Lab Animal*, 22 (8), 24, 1993.

106. Rehbinder, C;, Health Monitoring, in *Handbook of Laboratory Animal Science*, Vol. 1, Svendsen, P. and Hau, J. Eds., CRC Press, Boca Raton, 1994, 155.

107. Prasad, S., Gatmaitan, B. R., and O'Connell, R. C., Effect of a conditioning method on general safety test in guinea pigs, *Laboratory Animal Science*, 28, 591, 1978.

108. Clarke, G. L., Allen, A. M., Small, J. D., and Lock, A., Sub-clinical scurvy in the guinea pig, *Veterinary Pathology*, 17, 40, 1980.

109. Brewer, N. R. and Cruisee, L. J., Antioxidants simplified: Some species differences, Contemporary Topics in Laboratory Animal Science, 34, 92, 1996.

110. Nikkels, R. J. and Mullink, J. W. M. A., *Bordetella bronchiseptica* pneumonia in guinea pigs. Description of the disease and elimination by vaccination, *Zeitschrift fur Versuchstierkunde*, 13, 105, 1971.

111. Matherne, C. M., Steffen, E. K., and Wagner, J. E., Efficacy of commercial vaccines for protecting guinea pigs against *Bordetella bronchiseptica* pneumonia, *Laboratory Animal Science*, 37, 191, 1987.

112. Ganaway, J. R., Bacterial, mycoplasma and rickettsial diseases, in *The Biology of the Guinea Pig*, Wagner, J. E. and Manning, P.J. Eds., Academic Press, New York, 1976, 121.

113. Kohn, D. F., Bacterial otitis media in the guinea pig, *Laboratory Animal Science*. 24, 823, 1974.

114. Wagner, J. E. and Owens, D. R., Type XIX *Streptococcus pneumoniae (Diplococcus pneumoniae)* infections in guinea pigs, *Proceedings of the 21st Meeting of the American Association for Laboratory Animal Science*, Abstract No. 71, 1970.

115. Murphy, J. C., Ackerman, J. L., Marini, R.,P., and Fox, J. G., Cervical lymphadenitis in guinea pigs: Infection via intact ocular and nasal mucosa by *Streptococcus zooepidemicus*, *Laboratory Animal Science*, 41, 251, 1991.

116. Morris, T. H., Antibiotic therapeutics in laboratory animals, *Laboratory Animals*, 29, 16, 1995.

117. Rehg, J. E., Yarborough, B. A., and Pakes, S. P., Toxicity of cecal filtrates from gunea pigs with penicillin-associated colitis, *Laboratory Animal Science*, 30, 524, 1980.

118. Rehg, J. E. and Pakes, S. P., *Clostridium difficile* antitoxin neutralization of cecal toxin(s) from guinea pigs with penicillin-associated colitis, XXX 31, 156, 1981.

119. Seidl, D. C., Hughes, H. C., Bertolet, R., and Lang, C. M., True pregnancy toxemia (preeclampsia) in the guinea pig (*Cavia porcellus*), *Laboratory Animal Science*, 29, 472,1979.

120. Sauer, F., Fasting ketosis in guinea pigs, *Annals of the New York Academy of Science*, 104, 787, 1963.

121. Ganaway, R. J. and Allen, A. M., Obesity predisposes to pregnancy toxemia (ketosis) of guinea pigs, *Laboratory Animal Science*, 21, 40, 1971.

122. Bruss, M. L., Ketogenesis and ketosis, in *Clinical Biochemistry of Domestic Animals*, Laneko, J. J. Ed., Academic Press, San Diego, 1989, 86.

123. Olfert, E. D., Ward, G. E., and Stevenson, D., *Salmonella typhimurium* infection in guinea pigs: Observations on monitoring and control, *Laboratory Animal Science*, 26, 78, 1976.

124. Gentles, J. C., Experimental ringworm in guinea pigs: oral treatment with griseofulvin, *Nature (London)*, 182, 476, 1958.

125. McDonald, S. E. and Lavoipierre, M. M., *Trixacarus caviae* infestation in two guinea pigs, *Laboratory Animal Science*, 30, 67, 1980.

126. Harkness, J. E. and Wagner, J. E., Clinical Signs and Differential Diagnoses, in *The Biology and Medicine of Rabbits and Rodents,* Lea & Febiger, Philadelphia, Pennsylvania, 1989, 85.

127. Harkness, J. E. and Wagner, J. E., Specific Diseases and Conditions, in *The Biology and Medicine of Rabbits and Rodents,* Lea & Febiger, Philadelphia, Pennsylvania, 1989, 111.

128. Ediger, R. D., Warnick, C. L., and Hong, C. C., Malocclusion of the premolar and molar teeth in the guinea pig, *Laboratory Animal Science*, 25, 760, 1975.

129. Hurley, R. J., Murphy, J. C., and Lipman, N. S., Diagnostic Exercise: Depression and anorexia in recently shipped guinea pigs, Laboratory Animal Science, 45, 305, 1995.

130. Ellis, P. A. and Wright, A. E., Coccidiosis in guinea pigs, *Journal of Clinical Pathology*, 14, 394, 1961.

131. Shadduck, J. A. and Pakes, S. P., Encephalitozoonosis (nosematosis) and toxoplasmosis, *American Journal of Pathology*, 64, 657, 1971.

132. Wan, C.-H., Franklin, C. Riley, L. K., Hook, R. R., and Besch-Williford, C., Diagnostic Exercies: Granulomatous Encephalitis in guinea pigs, *Laboraotry Animal Science*, 46, 228, 1996.

133. Motzel, S. L. and Wagner, J. E., Diagnostic Exercise: Fetal death in guinea pigs, *Laboratory Animal Science*, 39, 341, 1989,

134. Van Hoosier, Jr., G. L., Giddens, Jr., W. E., Gillet, C. S., and Davis, H., Disseminated cytomegalovirus disease in the guinea pig, *Laboratory Animal Science*, 35, 81, 1985.

135. Kazdan, J. J., Schachter, J., and Okumoto, M. A., Inclusion conjunctivitis in the guinea pig, *American Journal of Ophthalmology*, 64, 116, 1967.

136. Fritz, P. E., Hurst, W. J., White, W. J., and Lang, C. M., Pharmacokinetics of cefazolin in guinea pigs, *Laboratory Animal Science*, 37, 646, 1987.

137. Hawk, C. T. and Leary S. L., Formulary for Laboratoy Animals, Iowa State University Press, Ames, 1995.

138. Harkness, J. E. and Wagner, J. E., Clinical Procedures, in *The Biology and Medicine of Rabbits and Rodents*, Lea & Febiger, Philadelphia, Pennsylvania, 1989, 55.

139. Dorrestein, G. M., Enrofloxicin in pet avian and exotic animal therapy, in *Proceedings of the 1st International Baytril Symposium*, Bonn: Bayer AG, 63, 1992.

140. Otto, C. M., Kaufman, G. M., and Crowe, D. T., Intraosseous infusion of fluids and therapeutics, *Compendium on Continuing Education for the Practicing Veterinarian*, 11 (4), 421, 1989.

141. Radde, G. R., Hinson, A., Crenshaw, D., and Toth, L. A., Evaluation of anesthetic regimens in guinea pigs, *Laboratory Animals*, 30, 220, 1996.

142. Brown, J. J., Thorne, P. R., and Nuttall, A. L., Blood pressure and other physiological responses in awake and anesthetized guinea pigs, *Laboratory Animal Science*, 39, 142, 1989.

143. Flecknell, P. A., Medetomidine and atipamezole: Potential uses in laboratory animals, *Lab Animal*, 26 (2), 21, 1997.

144. Strother, N. E. and Stokes, W. S., Evaluation of yohimbine and tolazoline as reversing agents for ketamine-xylazine anesthesia in the guinea pig, *Laboratory Animal Science*, 39, 482, 1989.

145. Flecknell, P. A., *Laboratory Animal Anesthesia*, Academic Press Limited, London, 1987.

146. Sawyer, D. C., *The Practice of Small Animal Anesthesia*, Major Problems in Veterinary Medicine, Vol. 1, W. B. Saunders Company, Philadelphia, 1982.

147. Barzago, M. M., Bortolotti, A., Stellari, F. F., Pagani, C., Marraro, G., and Bonati, M., Respiratory and hemodynamic functions, blood-gas parameters, and acid-base balance of ketamine-xylazine anesthetized guinea pigs, *Laboratory Animal Science*, 44, 648, 1994.

148. Parker, J. L. and Adams, J., R., The influence of chemical restraint agents on cardiovascular function: a review, *Laboratory Animal Science*, 28, 575, 1978.

149. Brewer, N. R. and Cruise, L. J., The respiratory systems of the guinea pig: Emphasis on species differences, *Contemporary Topics in Laboratory Animal Science*, 36, 100, 1997.

150. Blouin, A. and Cormier, Y., Endotracheal intubation in guinea pigs by direct laryngoscopy, *Laboratory Animal Science*, 37, 244, 1987.

151. Kujime, K. and Natelson, B. H., A method for endotracheal intubation of guinea pigs (*Cavia porcellus*), *Laboratory Animal Science*, 31, 715, 1981.

152. Levy, D. E., Zwies, A., and Duffy, T. E., A mask for delivery of inhalation gases to small laboratory animals, *Laboratory Animal Science*, 30, 868, 1980.

153. Franz, D. R. and Dixon, R. S., A mask system for halothane anesthesia of guinea pigs, *Laboratory Animal Science*, 38, 743, 1988.

154. Eisele, P. H., Kaaekuahiwi, M. A., Canfield, D. R., Golub, M. S., and Eisele, J. H., Epidural catheter placement for testing of obstetrical analgesics in female guinea pigs, *Laboratory Animal Science*, 44, 486, 1994.

155. Plumb, D. C., *Veterinary Drug Handbook*, 2nd ed., Iowa State University Press, Ames, 1995.

156. Morton, D. B. and Griffiths, P. H. M., Guidelines on the recognition of pain, distress, and discomfort in experimental animals and an hypothesis for assessment, *The Veterinary Record*, 116, 431, 1985.

157. Hubbell, J. A. E. and Muir, W. W., Evaluation of a survey of the diplomates of the American College of Laboratory Animal Medicine on use of analgesic agents in animals used in biomedical research, *Journal of the American Veterinary Medical Association*, 209, 918, 1996.

158. Romanovsky, A. A., Surgery in rodents: Risk of potential hypo- and hyperthermia, *AWIC Newsletter*, 4 (4), 7, 1993.

159. Gentry, S. J. and French, E. D., The use of aseptic surgery on rodents used in research, *Contemporary Topics in Laboratory Animal Science*, 33,6, 1994.

160. McCurnin, D. M. and Jones, R. L., Principles of surgical asepsis, in *Textbook of Small Animal Surgery*, Vol. 1, 2nd ed., Slatter, D. H, Ed., W. B. Saunders, Philadelphia, 1993, 114.

161. Brown, M. J., Pearson, P. T., and Tomson, F. N., Guidelines for animal surgery in research and teaching, *American Journal of Veterinary Research*, 54, 1544, 1993.

162. Cunliffe-Beamer, T. L., Applying principles of aseptic surgery to rodents, *AWIC Newsletter*, 4 (2), 1993.

163. Feldman, D. B. and Gupta, B. N., Histopathologic changes in laboratory animals resulting from various methods of euthanasia, *Laboratory Animal Science*, 26, 218, 1976.

164. Howard, H. L., McLaughlin-Taylor, E., and Hill, R. L., The effect of mouse euthanasia techniques on subsequent lymphocytic proliferation and cell mediated lympholysis assays, *Laboratory Animal Science*, 40, 510, 1990.

165. Butler, M. M., Griffey, S. M., Clubb, F. J., Gerrity, L. W., and Campbell, W. B., The effect of euthanasia technique on vascular arachidonic acid metabolism and vascular and intestinal smooth muscle contractility, *Laboratory Animal Science*, 40, 277, 1990.

166. AVMA Panel on Euthanasia, 1993 Report of the AVMA panel on euthanasia, *Journal of the American Veterinary Medical Association*, 202, 229, 1993.

167. Kesel, M. L., Handling, restraint, and common sampling and administration techniques in laboratory species, in *The Experimental Animal in Biomedical Research*, Vol. 1, Rollin, B. E. and Kesel, M. L. Eds., CRC Press, Boca Raton, 1990, 350.

168. McKeon, W. B., Jr., A critical evaluation of the antagonism of drugs to intravenous histamine in the guinea pig, *Archives of Internal Pharmacodynamic Therapy*, 141, 565, 1963.

169. Joint Working Group on Refinement, Removal of blood from laboratory mammals and birds, *Laboratory Animal*, 27, 1, 1993.

170. McGuill, M. W. and Rowan, A. N., Biological effects of blood loss: Implications for sampling volume and techniques, *ILAR News*, 31 (4), 5, 1989.

171. Hitzelberg, R., Lundgren, E., and Phillips, J., Guinea Pig, in *Laboratory Manual for Basic Biomethodology of Laboratory Animals*, Vol. 1, MTM Associated, Inc., Silver Springs, 1985, 3AI.

172. Reuter, R. E., Venipuncture in the guinea pig, *Laboratory Animal Science*, 37, 245, 1987.

173. Palumbo, N. E., Perrl, S. F., and Taylor, D., Guinea pig percutaneous femoral blood sampling technic using a new restraining device, *Laboratory Animal Science*, 25, 216, 1975.

174. Carraway, J. H. and Gray, L. D., Blood collection and intravenous injections in the guinea pig via the medial saphenous vein, *Laboratory Animal Science*, 39, 623. 1989.

175. Dolence, D. and Jones, H. E., Percutaneous phlebotomy and intravenous injections in the guinea pig, *Laboratory Animal Science*, 25, 106, 1975.

176. Decad, G. M. and Birnbaum, L. S., Noninvasive technique for intravenous injections of guinea pigs, *Laboratory Animal Science*, 31, 85, 1981.

177. Bullock, L. P., Repetitive blood sampling from guinea pigs (*Cavia porcellus*), *Laboratory Animal Science*, 33, 70, 1983.

178. Matolla, A. C., Eldridge, L., Herring, V. *et al.*, A comparison of passive cutaneous anaphylaxis guinea pig responses using an intravenous or an intradermal route for antigen challenge, *Journal of the American Oil Chemical Society*, 47, 458, 1970.

179. Lopez, H. and Navia, J. M., A technique for repeated collection of blood from the guinea pig, *Laboratory Animal Science*, 27, 522, 1977.

180. Srader, R. E. and Everson, G. J., Intravenous injection and blood sampling using cannulated guinea pigs, Laboratory Animal Care, 18, 214, 1968.

181. Sutherland, S. D. and Festing, M. F. W., The guinea-pig, in *The UFAW Handbook on The Care & Management of Laboratory Animals*, 6th ed., Poole, T. B., Ed., Churchill Livingstone, Inc. New York, 1987, 393.

182. Mandavilli, U., Schmidt, J., Rattner, D. W., Watson, W. T., and Warshaw, A. L., Continuous complete collection of uncontaminated urine in conscious rodents, *Laboratory Animal Science*, 41, 258, 1991.

183. Hoar, R. M., Biomethodology, in *The Biology of the Guinea Pig*, Wagner, J. E., and Manning, P.J. Eds., Academic Press, New York, 1976, 13.

184. Loizzi, R. F. and Guerin, M. A., Multiple biopsies of guinea pig mammary glands during pregnancy and lactation, *Laboratory Animal Science*, 29, 221, 1979.

185. Myers, S., Sparks, J. W., and Makowski, E. L., Factors affecting radioactive microsphere measurement of blood flow in pregnant guinea pigs, *Laboratory Animal Science*, 36, 522, 1986.

186. Liu, C.-T. and Guo, Z.-M., Cardiovascular responses to intracerebroventricular infusion of artificial cerebrospinal fluid in anesthetized strain 13 guinea pigs, *Laboratory Animal Science*, 42, 275, 1992.

187. Priekorn, D. M., Miller J. M., and Dolan, D. F., Reliable delivery system for chronic administration of substances into the inner ear of the guinea pig, *Contemporary Topics in Laboratory Animal Science*, 34, 65, 1995.

188. Kleinman, N,. R., Kier, A. B, Diaconu, E., and Lass, J. H., Posterior paresis induced by Freund's adjuvant in guinea pigs, *Laboratory Animal Science*, 43, 364, 1993.

189. Robuccio, J. A., Griffith, J. W., Chroscinski, E. A., Cross, P. J., Light, T. E., and Lang, C. M., Comparison of the effects of five adjuvants on the antibody response to influenza virus antigen in guinea pigs, *Laboratory Animal Science*, 45, 420, 1995.

190. Houston, L., Moncia, B. J., Page, R., and Engel, D., Response of guinea pigs to a vaccine containing a new adjuvant (SAF) and gram-negative bacteria, *Laboratory Animal Science*, 45, 59, 1995.

191. Ruble, D. L., Elliott, J. J., Wang, D. M., and Jaaz, G. P., A refined guinea pig model for evaluating delayed-type hypersensitivity reactions caused by Q fever vaccines, *Laboratory Animal Science*, 44, 608, 1994.

192. Heisey, G. B., Hughes, H. C., Lang, C. M., and Rozmiarek, H., The guinea pig as a model for isoniazid-induced reactions, *Laboratory Animal Science*, 30, 42, 1980.

193. CFR, Subpart E, 798.4100, Dermal Sensitization, *Health Effects Test Guidelines* as amended 1989, revised 1996, 172.

194. CFR, Subpart B, 610.11, *General Safety* as amended, revised 1996.

195. Magnusson, B. and Kligman, A. M., *Allergic Contact Dermatitis in the Guinea Pig*, Charles C Thomas, Springfield, 1970.

196. Buehler, E. V. and Ritz, H. L., Planning, conduct, and interpretation of guinea pig sensitization patch tests, *Cutaneous and Ocular Toxicity*, 28, 1980.

197. Jawetz, E., Melnick, J. L., and Adelberg, E. A., Immunology: II. Antibody-mediated and cell-mediated (hypersensitivity and immunity) reactions, in *Review of Medical Microbiology*, 11th ed., Lange Medical Publications, Los Altos, 1974, 163.

198. Swearengen, J. R., Cockman-Thomas, R. A., Davis, J. A., and Weina, P. J., Evaluation of butorphanol tartrate and buprenorphine hydrochloride on the inflammatory reaction of the Sereny test, *Laboratory Animal Science*, 43, 471, 1993.

199. Feldman, D. B. and Seely, J. C., *Necropsy Guide: Rodents and the Rabbit*, CRC Press, Inc., Boca Raton, 1988.

200. Formaldehyde Panel: Report of the Federal Panel on Formaldehyde, National Toxicology Program, Research Triangle Park, 1980.

index

AAALAC International, 50–51
Abortion, 25, 61, 64
Abscesses, 64, 65–66
Abyssinian Breed, 4, 5
Accreditation, 50–51, 52
Acepromazine, 82, 88, 111
Activity cycle, 6
Acute death, 61
Adjuvants, 121, 125
Ad libitum feeding and watering, 39, 41
Administration of drugs
  abbreviations used, 78, 81
  techniques, 110–121
Aggression, 8–9, 37
Air, recirculation of, 37
Albinos, 3
Albumin, 22
Allergies, 54
Alopecia, 61, 69–73
ALPHA, 133
Alpha male, 8, 9
Aluminum phosphate, 121
American Association for Laboratory Animal Science, 129–130
American Breed, 2, 3
American College of Laboratory Animal Medicine, 130

American Society of Laboratory Animal Practitioners, 130–131
Amino acids, 39
Analgesia, 81, 88–89
Anaphylaxis, 23
Anaphylaxis test, 125
Anatomy
  external, 9–10, 11
  internal, 10, 12–17
Anesthesia, 80–88
  four stages of, 90–91
  gas
    characteristics of, 86–87
    euthanasia by, 95
    principles of, 84–86
    suppliers, 136
  injectable, 81–84
  local, 87–88
Anesthetic care, 90–92
Anesthetic machine, 84
Animal care equipment, 29.
  See also Equipment
Animal care program, 41–42
Animal health
  monitoring, 55–56
  records, 47–48
Animal rooms, 28, 42, 43–45
Animal sources, 134–135

Animal Welfare Act, 27–28, 29,
    45, 49, 51, 53, 92
Animal Welfare Assurance, 50
Anterior vena cava, 101, 112
Antibiotics, 63, 65, 79
Antibiotic toxicity, 66
Anticoagulants, 79
Antigenicity test, 125
Antihelmentics, 79
Antihistamines, 79
Anus, 10, 11
Ascorbic acid, 39–40
Aseptic surgery, 92–93, 110
Aspirin, 89
Association for Assessment and
    Accreditation of Laboratory
    Animal Care International,
    Inc., 50–51, 130
Atipamezole, 83
Atropine, 83
Atropine sulfate, 82
Attend postures, 8
Aural administration, 120
Auricular veins, 107, 111
Automatic feeding devices, 34–35
Automatic watering devices,
    32–33, 42

"Baby fur," 69
Bacitracin, 66
Bacteria, 38, 46, 53–55
Barbering, 69
Basophils, 21
Bedding, 34, 38, 42
Behavior, 6–9
    coprophagic, 41
    group housing, 37
    during illness, 60
    introduction of novel items and,
        38
Bell jar, 86
Bibliography, 139–157
Biliary system, 14
Bilirubin, 22
Biologic parameters, 19
Biology of the Guinea Pig, The, 4
Birth weight, 24
Bladder, 17, 109

Blood, hematology, 19–22, 89
Blood collection, 99–109
Blood pH, 40
Blood pressure, 23
Blood urea, 22
Blood volume, 23, 99–100
Body heat, 91
Body surface area, 19
Body weight, 19, 24, 61
Books, reference, 132
Bordetella bronchiseptica, 61,
    62–64
Breeding
    cycle length, 24
    duration of, 24
    onset, 24
Breeding exhibitions and
        competition, 4
Breeds, 2–5
Bronchi, 15
Bronchopneumonia, 63
Buehler closed-patch
        sensitization test, 121,
        123–124
Bulbourethral glands, 16
"Bumblefoot," 77
Buprenorphine, 89
Butorphanol, 89

Cages, 30–35, 42–43, 136
Cage system, 32, 42
Cage washers, 43, 136
Calcium, 40
Carbon dioxide, 95
Cardiocentesis, 102–105
Cardiovascular function, 22–23,
    91, 92
Carotid artery, 107, 108, 109
Carriers, of disease, 63, 65
Catheters
    indwelling, 109, 113
    to inner ear, 120–121
Cavia procellus. See Guinea pigs
Cecum, 13, 14
Cefazolin, 79
Census, 48
Centers for Disease Control
        (CDC), 55

Central adrenergic neurons, 23
Cephalexin, 79
Cephalic vein, 107, 108
Cervical collar, 94, 136
Cervical lymphadenitis, 65–66
Cervical thymus. *See* Thymus
Cervix, 18
Chemicals
 for disinfection, 43
 occupational health and, 55
Chirodiscoides caviae, 71–72
Chlamydia psittaci, 54, 61, 78
Chloramphenicol, 63, 66
Chloramphenicolpalmitate, 79
Chloramphenicol succinate, 79
Chloresterol, 22
Chloride, 22
Chlorpromazine, 88
Chlortetracycline, 66
Chromosome number, 19
Circadian rhythms, 6
Citric acid, 43
Clavicles, 12
Clindamycin, 66
Clinical chemistry values, 22
Clotting factor values, 21
Coagulating glands, 16
Colon, 17
Colonies, behavior, 6
Coloration, 3, 47
Communication, 7–8
Comparative Medicine Discussion
 List, 133
COMPMED, 133
Compound administration
 techniques, 110–121
Conjunctivitis, 54, 61, 78
Coprophagic, 41
Copulatory plug, 24–25
Counters, 42
Creatinine, 22
Cryptosporidium, 54
Cryptosporidium wrairi, 74–75
Cytocentesis, 110
Cytomegalovirus, 75–76

Decapitation, 95
Defensive aggression, 8

Dehydration, 33, 61, 78, 80
Dentition, 10, 73–74
Dermatophytes, 54, 70
Descending colon, 17
Dexamethasone, 79
Diarrhea, 61
Diazepam, 82, 88
Diet, 39–41
Diphenylhydramine, 79
Disease, 53–55
 antibiotics for, 63, 65, 79
 clinical signs of, 60
 common, 61
 general treatment for, 78–80
 prevention procedures, 65, 80
 protozoal, 74–75
 viral, 75–77
Disinfection, 29, 80, 136
Documentation, 46–48
Doors, 29
Dorsolateral penile vein, 107, 108
Dosages
 abbreviations used, 78
 analgesics, 89
 euthanasia, 94–95
 general anesthetic agents, 82
 reversal agents, 83
 sedatives and tranquilizers, 88
Dosing needle, 118, 119
Doxapram, 83
Drainage, 28
Droperidol, 82, 84
Ductus deferens, 16
Duncan-Hartley strain, 2
Dyspnea, 63, 64

Ear notch, 47, 48
Ear pinch reflex, 91
Ears, 10, 59, 120–121
Ear tags, 47, 136
Eimeria caviae, 74–75
Electrocardiograms, 22
Electronic resources, 133–134
Elimination, behavior, 6
Encephalitozoon cuniculi, 75
Endotracheal tube, 84, 86
English Breed, 2, 3
Enrichment, 37–38

Enrofloxacin, 66, 79
Enteric bacteria, 66
Environmental conditions,
    35–37, 46
Environmental enrichment,
    37–38
Eosinophils, 21
EPA (U.S. Environmental
    Protection Agency), 50
Epididymis, 16, 18
Equipment
    animal care, 29
    cleaning, 29
    post-mortem examination,
        126
    protective, 43, 54, 55, 127
    research, 29
    sanitation procedures, 42
    suppliers, 135–138
    veterinary, 57–58
Erythrocytes, 20
Erythromycin, 66
Estrus, 24
Euthanasia, 94–95
Exhibitions and competition, 4
Experimental methodology,
    97–128
Eyes, Se also Conjunctivitis, 23,
    58, 90

Face mask, 84
Factor II, 21
Factor V, 21
Factor VIII, 21
Factor IX, 21
Fasting, 90
FDA (U.S. Food and Drug
    Administration), 50
Feces, 58, 78
Feed, 6
    containers, 34–35, 39
    limitations of rabbit food, 41
    novel food items, 38
    storage of, 40–41
    suppliers, 135
    transition to new diet, 39
    transit time through
        gastrointestinal system, 19

during transportation, 46
    unlimited, 39
    volume consumed per day, 19
Feet, 10, 58, 77
Females, 2
    body weight, 19
    breeding onset, 24
    milk collection, 110
    pregnancy toxemia, 67
    reproductiive function, 24–26
    reproductive behavior, 9
    reproductive organs, 16, 17
Femoral vessels, blood collection,
    107
Fentanyl, 82, 84
Fetuses, 25
Fiber, 39, 41
Fibrinogen, 21
Fleeing response, 6
Flight response, 6, 97
Floorplan, of laboratory facility,
    28
Floors, 28, 29
    of cages, 30–31
    sanitation procedures, 42
Footpad, 107, 108
Formaldehyde, 126
Formalin, 126
Fostering, 9
Freezing response, 6, 8
Freund's complete adjuvant
    (FCA), 121, 125
Fungal infections, 70

Gallbladder, 15
Gastrointestinal system, 14–15,
    19
General anesthesia, 81
Genotype, color, 3
Gentamicin, 79
Gestation, 24, 25, 67
Gestational alopecia, 69
Gliricola porcelli, 72, 73
Globulin, 22
Glycopyrrolate, 90
*Good Laboratory Practices for
    Nonclinical Laboratory
    Studies*, 50

Griseofulvin, 79
Grooming, 7
*Guide for the Care and Use of
    Laboratory Animals, The,*
    27, 29–30, 45, 50, 51, 53,
    92
Guinea pig antigenicity test,
    125
Guinea pigs, 2
  consumption of, 1
  identification, 47, 136
  origin of term, 2
  purpose-bred, 53
  sources, 55, 134–135
Gyropus ovalis, 72

Hair, 4, 58
  alopecia, 61, 69–73
  external parasites on, 70–73
  piloerection of, 8
Hairless guinea pigs, 4
Halothane, 82, 86
Handbook of Facilities Planning,
    27
Hartley strain 2, 2, 3
Hartley strain 13, 2, 3
Health Extension Act of 1985,
    50
Health records, 47–48
Heart, blood collection,
    102–105
Heart rate, 22, 23
Heat-sensitive temperature tape,
    43
Hematology, 19–22, 89
Hemoglobin concentration, 19,
    21
Hemolymphatic system, 12–14
Heparin, 79
Histamine sensitivity, 23
Histopathology, 46, 123
Historical background, 1–2
Holding technique, 97–99
Housing, 28
Humidity, 36
Husbandry, 27–48
Hydrogen ions, 40
Hypersensitivity reaction, 15

Hyperthermia, 61
Hypothermia, 61, 78, 80
Hypovolemic shock, 99

IACUC (Institutional Animal Care
    and Use Committee), 51–53
Ibuprofen, 89
Identification, 47, 136
ID (intradermal administration),
    116–117
Illumination, 36–37
IM (intramuscular
    administration), 113–114
Indwelling catheters, 109, 113
Infection. *See also* Antibiotics
  pathogens, 38, 53–55
  signs of, 93–94
Institute for Laboratory Animal
    Resources, 131
Institutional Animal Care and
    Use Committee (IACUC),
    51–53
International Council for
    Laboratory Animal Science,
    131
Intestinal disease, 54
Intracerebroventicular
    administration, 120
Intradermal administration (ID),
    116–117
Intramuscular administration
    (IM), 113–114
Intraperitoneal administration
    (IP), 115–116
Intravascular administration (IV),
    110–113
Intromittent sac, 16
IP (intraperitoneal
    administration), 115–116
Irritancy screening test, 123–124
Isoflurane, 82, 87
Ivermectin, 79
IV (intravascular administration),
    110–113

Jaw tone, 91
Jugular vein, 107, 108, 109
Juveniles, behavior, 9

Ketamine, 82, 83
Ketosis, 67
Kidney, 17
Kurloff cells, 20

Laboratory Animal Management
    Association, 131
Laboratory research
    databases, 133–134
    historical background, 1–2
    number used, 1994, 1
Lactation, 24, 25
Lameness, 61
Lateral metatarsal vein, 107, 112
Leukocytes, 21
Lidocaine, 87
Life span, 19
Lighting, 36–37
Lincomycin, 66
Listeria, 38
Litter size, 24
Liver, 14
Local anesthesia, 81, 87–88
Lungs, 15
Lymph nodules, 14
Lymphocytic choriomeningitis,
    76
Lymphocytres, 21
Lymphomyeloid complex, 20

Macroenvironment, 27, 36–37
Magnesium, 22, 40
Magnusson maximization test,
    121, 122–123
Males, 2
    body weight, 19
    breeding onset, 24
    reproductive behavior, 9
    reproductive function, 24–25
    reproductive organs, 16, 18
Malocclusion, 73–74
Mammae, 10
Management, 49–56
    animal care program, 41–42
    documentation, 46–48
    quality control program, 44
Manual manipulation, for urine
    collection, 109

Manual restraint, 97–99, 119
Marrow blood volume, 23
Masses/swelling, 61, 65–66, 75,
    123
Mating behavior, 8–9
Medial saphenous vein, 107,
    112
Meningeal disease, 53
Meperidine, 89
Metabolism cage, for urine
    collection, 109
Methohexital, 82, 83–84
Methoxyflurane, 82, 86–87
Metronidazole, 79
Microbiological monitoring,
    44–45
Microenvironment, 27, 37
Microsporum canis, 70
Milk collection, 110
Mineral requirements, 40
Monitoring
    animal health, 55–56
    animals during transporation,
        46
    commercial laboratories for,
        138
    microbiological, 44–45
    during postanesthetic care,
        92
    postsurgical, 93–94
Monocytes, 21
Morphine, 89
Mortality, 64
    acute death, 61
    antibiotic toxicity, 66
Mouth, 10, 59
Mucous membranes, color of, 91,
    92

Naloxone, 83
Nasal discharge, 63, 64
National Institutes of Health
    (NIH), 50
Necropsy, 46, 125–128, 136
Necrosis, 77
Needles
    for blood sampling, 102, 103,
        107

for drug administration, 111, 113, 114, 118, 119
suppliers, 136
Nesting materials, 38
Nests, lack of, 25
NETVET, 134
Network of Animal Health, 133
Neurologic disease, 61
Neutrophils, 21
NIH (National Institutes of Health), 50
NOAH online service, 133
Noise levels, 28, 37, 38
Nose cone, 8584
Nursing, 24, 26
Nutrition, 39–41

Occupational health, 53–55
Office for Protection from Research Risks (OPRR), 50
Olfactory signals, 7
One-stage prothrombin time (PT), 21
Online resources, 133–134
OPRR (Office for Protection from Research Risks), 50
Oral administration (PO), 118–120
Oral gavage, 118, 120
Organizations, 129–131
Osmotic pumps, 117, 136
Os penis, 11, 12
Ovaries, 16, 17
Oviducts, 16, 17
Ovulation, 24
Oxytetracycline, 66
Oxytocin, 79

Pain, indicators of, 88
Pancreatic duct, 15
Parasites
evaluation, 46
external, 70–73
Partial thromboplastin time (PTT), 21
Parturition, 9, 24, 25
Pathogens, 38, 46, 53–55. *See also* Disease; Parasites

Pedal reflex, 91
Pelvis, 12
Penicillin, 66
Penis, 11, 16
Pentobarbital, 82, 84, 95
Percutaneous blood sampling, 100–102, 108–109
Perianesthetic management, 89–92
Pericarditis, 64
Perineal sac, 10, 11
Perineum, 10, 11, 59
Periodicals, 132–133
Perivascular lymphoid nodules, 15
Personnel
interactions with, 38
occupational health, 53–55
protective equipment, 43, 54, 55, 127
surgical clothes, 93
work records of, 48
Peruvian Breed, 4
Peyer's patches, 14
Phenylbutazone, 89
Phosphoric acid, 43
Phosphorous, 40
PHS (Public Health Service), 50
Phylogeny, 2
Physical examination, 58–59, 89
Physiological features, 19–26
Piperazine salt, 79
Placenta, 25
Plasma volume, 23
Platelets, 21
Pleuritis, 64
Pneumonia, 38, 61, 62–65
Pododermatitis, 77
PO (oral administration), 118–120
Postanesthetic care, 92
Posterior vena cava, 103–104, 105
Post-mortem examination, 125–128
Postpartum estrus, 24
Postpartum pregnancy rate, 24
Postsurgical management, 93–94

Potassium, 22, 40
Preanesthetic care, 89–90
Precocial young, 19
Pregnancy rate, postpartum, 24
Pregnancy toxemia, 67
Prepuce, 11
Proestrus, 24
Proparacaine, 87–88
Prostate, 16, 18
Protective equipment, 43, 54, 55, 127
Proteins, 39, 41
Prothrombin, 21
Protozoal disease, 74–75
PT (one-stage prothrombin time), 21
PTT (partial thromboplastin time), 21
Publications, 132–133
Public Health Service (PHS), 50
Public Health Service Policy on Humane Care and Use of Laboratory Animals, 50, 52, 53, 92
Purpose-bred guinea pigs, 53, 89

Quality control program, 44
Quarantine, 59–60

Range, 2
Record keeping, 46–48
Red blood cells, 19–20, 21
References, 139–157
Reflexes, 91–92
Registration of facility, 49
Regulations of the Animal Welfare Act, 27–28, 29, 45, 49, 52, 53
Regulatory agencies, 49–53
Relative humidity, 36
Renal pelvis, 15
Renal tubules, 15
Report of the American Veterinary Medical Association Panel on Euthanasia, 94
Reproduction, 23–26
  behavior, 8–9

infertility from blockage by bedding, 35
similarities with humans, 23
Research, equipment, 29
Resources, 129–138
Respiratory disease, 53, 54
Respiratory rate, 23, 59, 91, 92
Respiratory system, 15
Restraint, 97–99, 119, 136
Retro-orbital sinus, blood collection, 105–107
Reversal agents, 83
Ribs, 12
Ringer's solution, 90
Ringworm, 54, 70
RODAC plates, 45
Routes of administration, 78, 81

Safety testing procedures, 121–125
Salmonella, 38
Salmonella dublin, 68
Salmonella enteriditis, 68
Salmonella typhimurium, 68
Salmonellosis, 67–69
Sampling techniques, 99–110
Sampling vials, 100
Sanitation, 41–45, 136
  disease prevention through, 65, 80
  equipment, 28
  procedures, 29
Scent, 7
Scrotal swelling, 11
SC (subcutaneous administration), 114–115
Scurvy, 61–62
Sedation, 81, 88
Sensitization tests, 121–125
Sensory enrichment, 38
Sereny test, 125
Serology, 46, 76
Serum
  clinical chemistry values, 22
  sampling, 100
Serum calcium, 22
Serum glucose, 22
Serum phosphate, 22

Serum protein, 22
Shigella, 125
Shipping container, 46
Sink, 28, 42
Skeletal system, 10, 12
Skin wounds, 53, 54
Sleep cycle, 6
Small intestine, 14
Smell, sense of, 7
Social behavior, 7–8
Sodium, 22
Sodium lauryl sulfate, 122
Spleen, 12
Stampeding response, 6, 97
Stand-threats, 8
Steroid resistance, 21
Stomach, 14
Streptococcus pneumoniae, 38, 61, 64–65
Streptococcus zooepidemicus, 65
Streptomycin, 66
Stress response, noise levels and, 28
Subcutaneous administration (SC), 114–115
Subcutaneous transponders, 47
Sulfamethazine, 75, 79
Sulfaquinoxaline, 79
Surface area of body, 19
Surgery
  aseptic, 92–93
  for urine collection, 110
Survival, 19
Swelling. *See* Masses/swelling
Symphysis, 12, 25

Tags, 47, 136
Tattoos, 47
Teeth, 10, 73–74
Temperature
  of animal room, 36, 80
  of guinea pig, 59, 91
Temperature tape, 43
Testes, 16, 18
Tetracycline, 79
Thoracic cavity, 13, 59
Thoracic inlet, 101

Thrombin time, 21
Thymus, 12, 13, 14, 20
Thyroxine, 22
Tidal volume, 23
Tiletamine, 82
Toes, 10
Torticollis, 61
Toxicity testing, 116
Toxoplasmosis, 61
Toys, 38
Tracheitis, 63
Tranquilization, 81, 88
Transportation, 45–46
Trehalose dimycolate, 121
Trichophyton mentagrophytes, 70
Triglycerides, 22
Triiodothyroxine, 22
Trimethoprim, 79
Trixacarus caviae, 54, 72, 73
Tumors. *See* Masses/swelling

Ureters, 15
Urethal orifice, 10, 11, 16
Urinary bladder, 17, 109
Urine, 19, 58, 78
Urine collection, 109–110
Urogenital system, 15–18
U.S. Department of Agriculture (USDA), 49
U.S. Environmental Protection Agency (EPA), 50
U.S. Food and Drug Administration (FDA), 50
USDA (U.S. Department of Agriculture), 49
Uterus, 16, 17

Vaccinations, 63
Vagina, 10, 11, 16, 17
Vaginal closure membrane, 11, 24
Vaginal cytology, 24
Veins
  blood collection and catheter sites, 107
  for drug administration, 112

Vendors, 55
Ventilation, 37
  during quarantine, 59
  during transportation, 46
Vertebral column, 12
Vesicular glands, 16
Veterinary care, 57–95
Veterinary supplies, 57–58
Vials, 100
Vibrissae, 10
Viral disease, 75–77
Vitamin C, 39–40, 61–62
Vitamin requirements, 39–40, 41
Vocalization, 7–8

Water consumption
  during transportation, 46
  unlimited, 41
  volume per day, 19

Watering devices, 31–33
  sanitation procedures, 42
Weaning age, 24, 26
Weight, 19, 24
Weight loss, 61
Whiskers, 10
Work records, 48

Xylazine, 82, 83, 88

Yohimbine, 83
Young
  at birth, 25
  nursing by, 25
  precocial, 9

Zolazepam, 82
Zoonotic disease, 69, 72, 76, 127
Zygomatic arch, 10

notes

notes

notes

notes

notes

notes

notes

notes

notes